Healing Hands by Dominique Giniaux
Copyright © 1998 by Xenophon Press

Original French edition © 1992 by Editions Lamarre, Paris.

Illustrations by Author

Translated by Jean-Claude Racinet

All rights reserved. No part of this work may be reproduced or transmitted in any form or by any means, electronic or mechanical, including photocopying, or by any information storage or retrieval system except by a written permission from the publisher.

Published by Xenophon Press LLC

7518 Bayside Road, Franktown, Virginia 23354-2106, U.S.A.

print edition
ISBN-10   0933316127
ISBN-13   9780933316126

e-book edition
ISBN-10:   0933316526
ISBN-13:   9780933316522

Cover design by Naia E. Poyer

HEALING HANDS

A TREATISE ON FIRST-AID EQUINE ACUPRESSURE

by DOMINIQUE GINIAUX, D.V.M.

With a Preface

By DR. JEAN PLAINFOSSE

Translated to English

By JEAN-CLAUDE RACINET

© Xenophon Press 1998

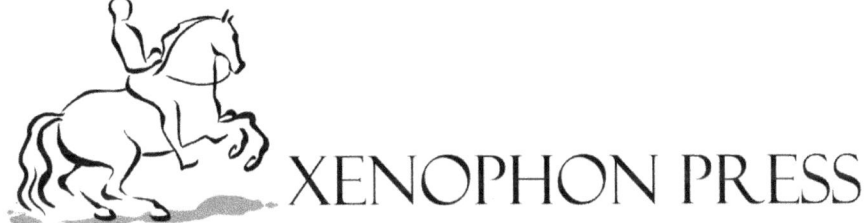

Xenophon Press Library

Xenophon Press continues to bring new works to print in the English language whether they be new works, such as this, or translations of older works. Xenophon Press is dedicated to the preservation of classical equestrian literature.
Available at www.XenophonPress.com

30 Years with Master Nuno Oliveira, Michel Henriquet 2011
A Rider's Survival from Tyranny, Charles de Kunffy 2012
Another Horsemanship, Jean-Claude Racinet, 1994
Art of the Lusitano, Yglesias de Oliveira, 2012
Baucher and His School, General Decarpentry 2011
Dressage in the French Tradition, Dom Diogo de Bragança 2011
École de Cavalerie Part II, François Robichon de la Guérinière 1992
François Baucher: The Man and His Method, Baucher/Nelson, 2013
Gymnastic Exercises for Horses Volume II, Eleanor Russell 2013
H. Dv. 12 Cavalry Manual of Horsemanship, Reinhold 2014
Healing Hands, Dominique Giniaux, DVM 1998
Horse Training: Outdoors and High School, Etienne Beudant 2014
Legacy of Master Nuno Oliveira, Stephanie Millham 2013
Methodical Dressage of the Riding Horse, Faverot de Kerbrech 2010
Racinet Explains Baucher, Jean-Claude Racinet 1997
The Art and Science of Riding in Lightness, Stodulka 2014
The Art of Traditional Dressage, Volume I DVD, de Kunffy 2013
Great Horsewomen of the 19th Century in the Circus, Nelson 2001
The Ethics and Passions of Dressage Expanded Ed., de Kunffy 2013
The Gymnasium of the Horse, Gustav Steinbrecht 2011
The Italian Tradition of Equestrian Art, Tomassini 2014
The Maneige Royal, Antoine de Pluvinel 2010
The Portuguese School of Equestrian Art, de Oliveira/da Costa, 2012
The Spanish Riding School & Piaffe and Passage, Decarpentry 2013
Total Horsemanship, Jean-Claude Racinet 1999
Wisdom of Master Nuno Oliveira, Antoine de Coux 2012

Available at www.XenophonPress.com

PREFACE

Dr. Giniaux has opened a door. He started drafts. That is what happens most to those who walk off the trodden paths.

This unconventional approach to the equine pathology and therapy has earned the right to be considered, as one can judge from the technical and psychological tests I put it through. Good results have been thus obtained.

I therefore made it my duty to encourage him to persevere in the direction he took, and which is already well received by the horse professionals.

Dr. Jean Plainfosse, Veterinarian
Crèvecoeur en Auge on July 26, 1986.

"For the thinking man, the apex of happiness lies in understanding what can be understood and to respect what cannot."
Goethe

INTRODUCTION

This is not about a crash course in acupuncture allowing to master in one or two hours this millennial art. Acupuncture is a form of therapy that one cannot pretend mastering correctly but after several years of study and practice. In the course of these studies, the only thing one understands very soon is that it will be impossible ever to consider oneself to be perfectly competent in this field. All its laws are fluid, as it goes for life itself, which is characterized by the fact that nothing is immutable in it.

The technique I am discussing gives us the opportunity to possibly check serious problems with the horse by using in a simple fashion some of the effects of acupuncture. Hence, in each case presented, these are specific recipes which have proven effective in many cases. All the data which you will find in this book were verified through the described protocol. They are not the theoretical deductions of an acupuncturist who would have contended himself by putting into writing some more elaborate methods, but rather a result from practices implemented as shown in the book.

Because of his hypersensitive nervous system, and a high tendency to display spasm phenomena, a horse is the ideal subject to this type of treatment. Results come up more rapidly with the horse than with the human, which easily contradicts those who argue of an action based on the "placebo" effect.[1]

---

[1] One calls "placebo effect" the fact that a patient is healed through an otherwise inoperative treatment which he or she has been persuaded will work. The success of acupuncture in the colics of horses can even not be explained by the fact that the animal understands one is taking care of him, since the same applies for classical medicine and the results are slower with the later.

This method must not be considered as one that would allow one not to call for the help of a veterinarian, but rather as a way to prevent the horse from suffering as he is waiting for him to arrive, even if very often your intervention was sufficient for a return to normalcy.

One must also be aware of the fact that, as with acupuncture itself, this therapeutic method puts demands on the energy reserves of the patient. Consequently, it requires from the organism sufficient strength to react, which it can do only if it is not exhausted by the disease, or by a poor general state.

Although some ill informed veterinarians or physicians state that "if acupuncture is worthless, it has at least the merit of doing no harm," one has to be aware that it can precipitate the end of a debilitated animal, or an animal in the state of serious shock.

If the method I am proposing to you is correctly applied, in its techniques as in its indications, you are going to be fully satisfied with the undeniable results it will often bring about, you will even be surprised with its rapidity of action in the case of some afflictions where the official approach has taught us to be patient.

In the field of colic, in particular, nobody is going to reproach you for having waited too long before calling the veterinarian, since you will know within ten to twenty minutes if your action was effective. When you are familiarized with this way of treatment, there will even be cases when the digestive transit will be reestablished during your intervention!

For the possible skeptics, I will simply add that considering the serious risk involved in any colic, denigrating and rejecting a new possibility of treatment without thoroughly trying it, amounts to setting little store by the life of a horse.

Read carefully what follows. That this method is relatively easy to implement does not mean that it is not very precise. More and more persons use it with satisfaction, and there is no reason why you could not do the same if you apply it scrupulously.

The second part of the book will offer you an insight into a somewhat identical technique, however based on a different theory of acupuncture, auriculotherapy. Here again, you will be offered a range of possibilities, ignored by many to this day.

The author

Contents

Preface   iii
Introduction   v

FIRST PART

ACUPUNCTURE   1
Chapter 1   3
Chapter 2
   Principles of Treatment   7
Chapter 3
   Recognizing and Treating the Points   13
Chapter 4
   Topography of the Points   17
Chapter 5
   Equine Colic   21
Chapter 6
   Ovary Problems   39
Chapter 7
   Foaling   45
Chapter 8
   Chronic Pulmonary Emphysema   57
Chapter 9
   Wind Sucking   61
Chapter 10
   Hyperhidrosis   63
Chapter 11
   Paroxysmal Myoglobinuria   65
Chapter 12
   Hemorrhages   71
Chapter 13
   Heat Stroke   75

Chapter 14
    Shoulder Lameness   77
Chapter 15
    Agitation   81

SECOND PART

AURICULOTHERAPY   85
Chapter 1   87
Chapter 2
    Historic Review   89
Chapter 3
    Mode of Action   93
Chapter 4
    Topography   95
Chapter 5
    Technique   99
Chapter 6
    Conclusion   104
Summary Chart   107

FIRST PART

ACUPUNCTURE

Chapter 1

Without dwelling on details, we have to say a few words on the bases of traditional acupuncture, if only to explain to what extent the techniques hereunder described part from it.

Traditional acupuncture is based essentially on the existence of a form of Energy which runs in a given number of well-defined circuits in any living organism.

To be an acupuncturist consists in knowing thoroughly the topography of these circuits, in appreciating perfectly the quantity and quality of the Energy which runs in them at the moment of the exam of the individual to be treated, finally in being capable of bringing back to normalcy the distribution of this Energy by choosing among several procedures; this choice depends on the individual, his/her actual state, his/her previous pathological history, and his/her environment (life conditions, current season, and even time of day for the exam, etc...).

The most commonly used means are stings by very fine needles, moxas (treatment of some points through an intense and brief heat), massage of precise points or lines, momentary compression of several points in a predetermined order, etc. Subsequently, one should be capable of appreciating the modifications introduced to the whole of the organism.

All this is far from being simple, as we see, and an obvious consequence stands out: there cannot be any therapeutic guide of acupuncture in the way we mean it in Western medicine. Such a guide, indeed, is a list of diseases, giving each of them the treatment to apply. It would be foolish to inventory the diseases that acupuncture can treat. This Chinese medicine does not treat any disease, it re-equilibrates the perturbed organisms and when it reaches this goal, the first consequence is the disappearance of the oncoming diseases; if this is not the result, it means that the equilibrium has still not been attained.

The Chinese tradition distinguishes several forms of energy and classifies the circuits in several more or less important networks. The more accessible energy runs through a succession of carefully itemized courses which are the main meridians. These twelve meridians take turns in a twenty-four hour cycle of conveying the Energy they are passing on. Each meridian, being loaded with the Energy for a two hour period daily, is therefore capable of assuring the function imparted to it of regulating all the organs concerned in any way with this meridian.

Each meridian contains an alignment of points among which one can distinguish:

• Five points allowing one to play with the distribution of the Energy; depending on the point and the way it is treated, one can slow the Energy down, accelerate it, deviate it toward another advisedly chosen meridian, or on the contrary attracts this which stagnates in an overloaded meridian.
• A sixth point, the so-called Tsri point, indicated in the acute afflictions of the principal organ which the meridian is named after, and sometimes in the afflictions situated on a territory through which this meridian is running.
• Although not situated on the meridian "per se," a seventh point whose function is essential. It is the Shu point, situated along the vertebral column. To each meridian corresponds a Shu point whose foremost function is to regulate the corresponding circuit, irrespective of the direction of its imbalance.

Considering this role of the Shu point, one understands why it is situated in the area where the autonomic nerves governing the same function stem from the spinal cord. One understands also why it is the main element of a method for standardized treatments such as this of which we are going to speak.

On this basis, it is possible to treat numerous cases through the Shu point corresponding to the ongoing affliction; it is often useful to add to it other points whose specific action is indicated for the cases it pertains to.

The success of such treatment, when it materializes, is very rapid. Therefore insisting stubbornly would be stupid and dangerous. Moreover, it is obvious that for the affliction which can be treated through a proven classical treatment, efficiently and giving quick results, engaging in such trials without knowing acupuncture would be illogical.

Chapter 2

PRINCIPLES OF TREATMENT

As previously stated, the Shu points will be used the most, because they are located where the autonomic fibers stem out of the nervous system. It is indeed the possibility of an action on the autonomic fibers which is the base of the method of treatment presented; to explain this, we must first describe in a few words the role of the autonomous system.

Every organ, with the living being, contributes to the functioning of the whole: for this, it should itself work correctly and furthermore should adapt to the surrounding conditions. Any organ whatsoever (heart, lung, intestine, or even the smallest blood vessel) does not function with the same intensity whether the individual is resting or makes an effort, is digesting or not, is quiet or stressed.

All these variations are taken in charge by the sympathetic and parasympathetic nervous system, also called the autonomic nervous system because it works mechanically, without the will of the individual.

By and large, every organ gets two kinds of autonomic nerves. One is meant for accelerating its functioning, the other for slowing it. One distinguishes the sympathetic fibers and the other the parasympathetic fibers, which are antagonistic to each other; they are in charge of controlling each other's excesses.

This mechanism of regulation corresponds precisely to the notion of Yin and Yang of the Chinese who hold that life and all the universe result from oscillations between two opposite forces.

When an organ is ailing, its autonomic innervation is out of balance on one way or the other, irrespective of the cause of the trouble. The imbalance provoked the disease or the disease provoked the imbalance, but the result is the same; the organism can heal only when the autonomic system starts oscillating again round the point of equilibrium.

The stimulation of the Shu point shakes the autonomic system of the corresponding organ, which comes to the same thing as shaking a blocked scale to allow it to oscillate anew freely.

One thus reactivates the beam of regulation of the organ where the trouble lies. The difference with numerous classical treatments is that these latter content themselves with pushing this beam way out in the direction opposite to its blocking. There usually comes about a reverse blocking and it takes time for the organism to react against these excesses. One understands thence why drugs so often result in a reversal of symptoms, while the real healing is lingering. Thus, many constipations treated in a classical way are succeeded by a diarrhea, then by an alternation between these two extremes, which ebbs progressively. We are indeed in the presence of a "pendulum" phenomenon, which confirms what I said of the mode of regulation by the autonomous system. This explains why too strong a medication can sometimes block the pendulum to the other side and why the final healing is slower with the allopathic drugs. Obtaining a brutal diarrhea after a constipation is still not healing: just look at the general state of the patient at this moment! His/her entourage are reassured by this opposite symptom, but the goal is not met.

To take care of a patient, I think it useful to have some understanding of the mode of action of the means at hand. If one can proceed from a reasoning one understands well, then one is able to chose the method most indicated for each case. By using a comparison drawn from a realm everybody knows, one may find a way amongst others of explaining life, health, disease through its different stages, and understand by and large where and how the means of classical medicine work. By correctly assessing in this picture the level of action of the method I propose, one will be able to clearly apprehend its limits and acknowledge its indications.

Let's compare the functioning of an organ—and even life itself—to a person who rides a bicycle on a straight line; whatever s/he does, the wheels will never trace a straight line on the ground. To understand that a straight line is possible only through permanent waves, one just has to try and ride on a bike whose front wheel has been blocked in a fore and aft position: one inevitably falls and one does not doubt anymore that balance cannot exist without slight, constantly compensated deviations on both sides of an imaginary line. The cessation of the functioning of the autonomic nervous system (i.e., the cessation of the antagonism Yin - Yang) is immediately followed with death. If this cessation concerns only one organ, this latter will rapidly be unable to carry out its mission and will jeopardize the whole of the organism.

The fall of a biker can happen in another way. If the oscillations become visible and more and more obvious, balance becomes very precarious and the individual has more difficulties in following the intended path; s/he is in real danger of ending up in the ditch. For a living organism, this process is a more frequent cause of death than the pure and simple cessation of the oscillations.

The biker's loss of balance can have several causes. It can be simply fatigue but also often an unexpected event: a patch of black ice, a chicken crossing the road, or a sudden fear, even unjustified. A tire puncture or a breaking down of a part of the bike are also possible causes for the fall but may sometimes proceed from some brutal and excessive swerving: the part which then breaks down is the most fragile and therefore that which has been too roughly handled or abnormally stressed.

To avoid the fall of the biker, there are several means which depend on the ongoing problem. One can restore his forces if he was too tired, shout at him to help him sit up if he was unaware of his deviating, limit quietly his deviation with one's shoulder when one rides besides him/her (it's risky), push bluntly his handlebars in the opposite direction (it's becoming really dangerous!), chase away the chicken about to cross the road, finally have him/her dismount from the bike to repair the fragile or already broken down part, if possible before the catastrophe happens.

It is important to mention that except in the case of a mechanical breakdown, the coming back into balance *is less risky if one urges the person to take charge himself/herself than if one intervenes in his/her place;* there are even cases when the biker deviates on purpose to avoid an obstacle we have not seen and it would then be wrong to set him back by force in the right way. In this case it is better to shout "watch out" to make sure s/he knows what s/he is doing.

This simple story of the bike that everybody can understand explains much in medicine.

By working essentially at the level of the "Shu" points, the mode of treatment which I am proposing to you calls the autonomic system to order where it is losing its balance, so that, through a reflex due to this call, it can resume its regular oscillations; *such a return will happen only if it is possible, therefore if the organ it belongs to has no lesions.* It won't happen as well if the deviation is only momentary and programmed by the organism facing an unexpected event. As it is, for instance, in the case of a reflex of diarrhea aimed at eliminating a food intoxication (like the biker who deviates momentarily in order to avoid a puddle).

Continue yourself the comparison and you'll see that it is therefore the first technique to try when facing a disease known for the important participation of the nervous system, like equine colic, myoglobinuria, ovary problems, urinary spasms, etc.

All these afflictions are very often not caused by a lesion, and the efficacy of the treatment is henceforth practically assured and very quick. And if it doesn't work, no time will have been wasted before using more classical means.

All this is not about acupuncture properly speaking since we haven't had to take into account the distribution of the Energy, which an acupuncturist knows how to assess and modify with precision. However, we will sometimes use points other than the Shu points.

Their action often has a complex energetic explanation for each point but cannot be reduced to a reflex of the nervous system.

Although the treatments hereunder described are recipes categorized by affliction, the basic theory of acupuncture will be partly respected. Indeed, it will be about treating individuals and not diseases because, although starting from a common basis, the treatments will be in each case individualized. You will have to learn how to chose among a list of points which fit not only the case, but also the horse on that day. You will have to learn how to check all the points concerned and discern through palpation those which must be treated.

Coming now to the technique itself, let us start with learning how to check a point.

Chapter 3

RECOGNIZING AND TREATING THE POINTS

Describing a sensation is not easy, but there is no other way to learn how to localize a point on the horse you are presented with, and feel whether it must be treated or not.

The localization "per se" is a relatively simple topographical question which requires only a few diagrams. As you are progressing in your research, you will rapidly notice that acupuncture points are always situated in a depression which is easy to feel with the finger even if sometimes it is not visible; this depression is the size of a finger tip and it is therefore what is to be looked for in the concerned area.

Then one must check every point concerned with the ongoing affliction and thus decide if it must be treated; this not only allows one to diagnose the ailing organs, but will also individualize the treatment by modifying the basic "recipe" according to the patient.

A sound, balanced point and therefore unrelated to the case at hand is normally supple and its pressure by the finger does not entail any local reaction; I underline "local," because one should not take into account the fact that the horse turns his neck or tries to kick or starts any other movement of defense. Such a general reaction is due to the ticklish character of the animal, his being upset by the troubles which afflict him, and essentially by his feeling we are nearing the sensitive area, the diverse points being sometimes close to one another.

To be able to affirm that a point responds to the pressure test, one must feel at once a local abnormal tension and the pressure must provoke an immediate reflex of contraction of the subcutaneous muscles. One gets accustomed very quickly to appreciating these nuances, according to the horse one intends to examine.

It is important to know how to recognize a pathologic point all the more as one will feel it become supple and normal during the treatment itself. Indeed, if the massage is correctly carried out, one observes a noticeable release under the finger within a few minutes, while the internal spasm relaxes and the corresponding function resumes. In the case of impaction colic in particular, it is often when you feel the most tense point yield under your finger tip that you will hear the first contraction of the bowel showing the resumption of the intestinal transit.

It is absolutely necessary to check several times a point in the course of a treatment and more so in the end, since it may happen that we have "displaced" the problem of the horse; another organ may in turn react whereas it was not concerned in the beginning. One must then treat this new problem which is always less serious; it is somehow a step toward the healing which would have resolved of its own but which can be helped in this way, all the more easily as a favorable response was just being given by the organism.

The behavior of a horse in the course of a treatment shows very well that he is sensitive to what is happening; he first tries to shy off of your action, then he looks like he is accepting it, whereas in fact he is too preoccupied by his internal problem which seems to confirm itself first, then culminates before yielding. It is not rare that during all this time the horse turns his head toward you, observing what you are doing; even if he does not like it too much, he lets you come closer to him in the course of a session, whereas the sight of a syringe would rather make him cower into the back of his stall. I'm not trying to make the picture prettier to tell you a fairy tale, you'll see by yourself.

The treatment of the points will start with those which seem less affected. They will relax very quickly and you will proceed on to the next ones.

Apart from one or two points which I will indicate in due time, all those you will have to treat are symmetrically placed on the horse's body; therefore, *when I indicate a point, it should be localized, checked, and treated on both sides of the horse before passing on to the following.*

As for the technique itself, this which we are going to adopt is the easier to implement, whatever the context, since it does not require any material: it is a particular massage with the finger. Thus you will be able to treat in the middle of a field, on a trail, or anywhere, without further ado.

One also can treat with a brush on the area around the point, with the "prune tree flower hammer" of the Chinese which works with repeated stings, with a minute intradermal injection of water from a "Dermo-Jet," or finally, of course, with an acupuncture needle. These techniques do not dispense one from checking the point with a finger and are often more complicated, so let's limit ourselves to the technique which checks the point while it treats it and allows us to remain constantly aware of the situation.

You won't do a massage properly speaking, since your finger will not have rubbed the skin. *One should press rather strongly and rotate the tip of the finger as if one wanted to penetrate into the subcutaneous tissues through the skin;* it therefore is the skin, fixed by the finger, which moves over the muscles.

The Chinese say that in order to "disperse" a point, which is our purpose, it is better to rotate counterclockwise. I think that for these points, this is of rather little importance, and that one's finger gets less tired by changing direction from time to time. For a given point, one will generally treat the two sides of a horse successively (or simultaneously if the localization allows it and if one has long arms).

If the horse is nervous and likely to kick, it is better to keep a hand leaning against the hip: in the event the horse wants to turn his rear end or kick with a hind leg, one would be immediately pushed away by his gesture. Even a soft animal can start the gesture, particularly in a colic when the transit resumes. This precaution is absolutely necessary while treating ovary pains with a mare. The point of the ovaries being situated toward the upper part of the flank, one treats the right side of the mare with the right hand while leaning with the left hand onto the right hip and conversely.

When a point has been treated correctly, it does not react any more to the test. During the action of the finger, one has the impression that it sinks in as if one were softening a small zone of the underlying muscles; subsequently, the movement of the finger becomes easier.

Chapter 4

TOPOGRAPHY OF THE POINTS

The position of each point will be described in the practical part of this book as it unfolds, but let us first speak of the Shu points since they are more important and since the technique for seeking them is practically the same for all of them.

The Shu points are for the most part situated between the ribs, on the edge of the common mass of the dorsal muscles; each one will be defined through the intercostal space in which it lies, and therefore one will have to count the ribs from rear to front, starting from the hollow area of the flank, next to the hip. Let your finger run along the horse's side without pressing too strongly, but strongly enough anyway to feel clearly each rib (Fig. 1). When you have arrived at the space indicated for the Shu point you are looking for, direct your finger toward the vertebral column and push up between the two ribs, pressing a little more firmly in order to stay in the interval they define; you will end up infallibly in the depression where the Shu point is situated. It is precisely where your finger sinks in as it bumps against the edge of the dorsal common muscular mass (Fig.2).

At the level of the lumbar vertebrae (the loins) the points are in the middle of the muscular mass, on a line at mid-distance between the edge of the common mass and the top of the vertebral column (Fig. 3). We will anyway need only one of these points; it lies 8 to 10cm. (3 or 4 inches) back from the last rib on this line (Shu point of the small intestine).

The diagrams and photographs in the following pages illustrate these somewhat complicated explanations. Don't forget that the Shu

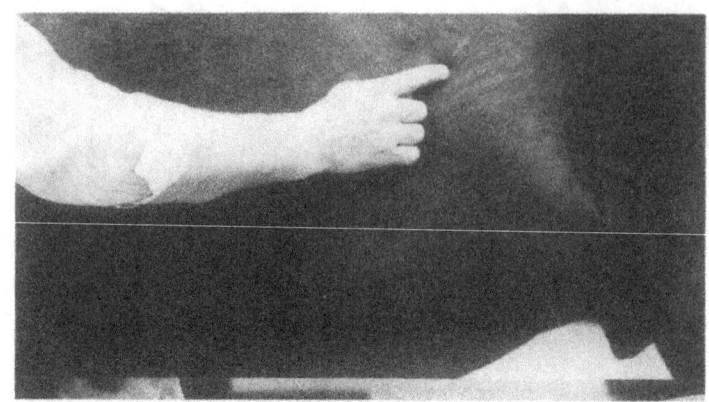

Fig. 1

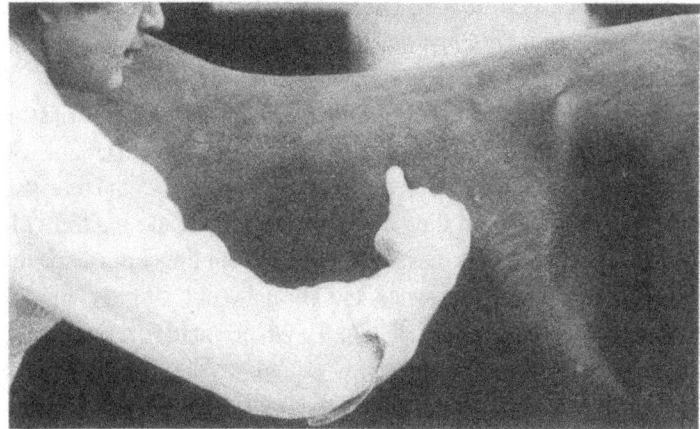

Fig. 2

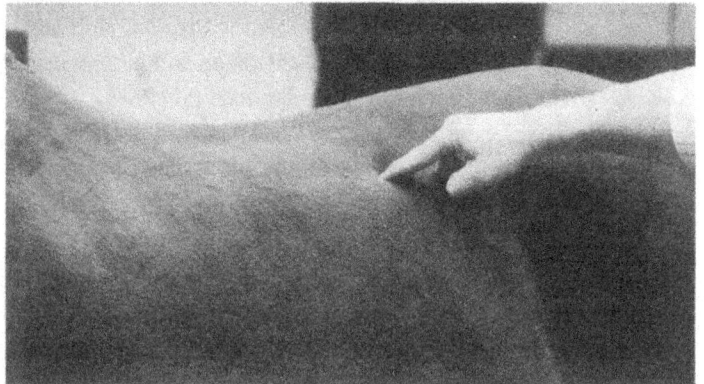

Fig. 3

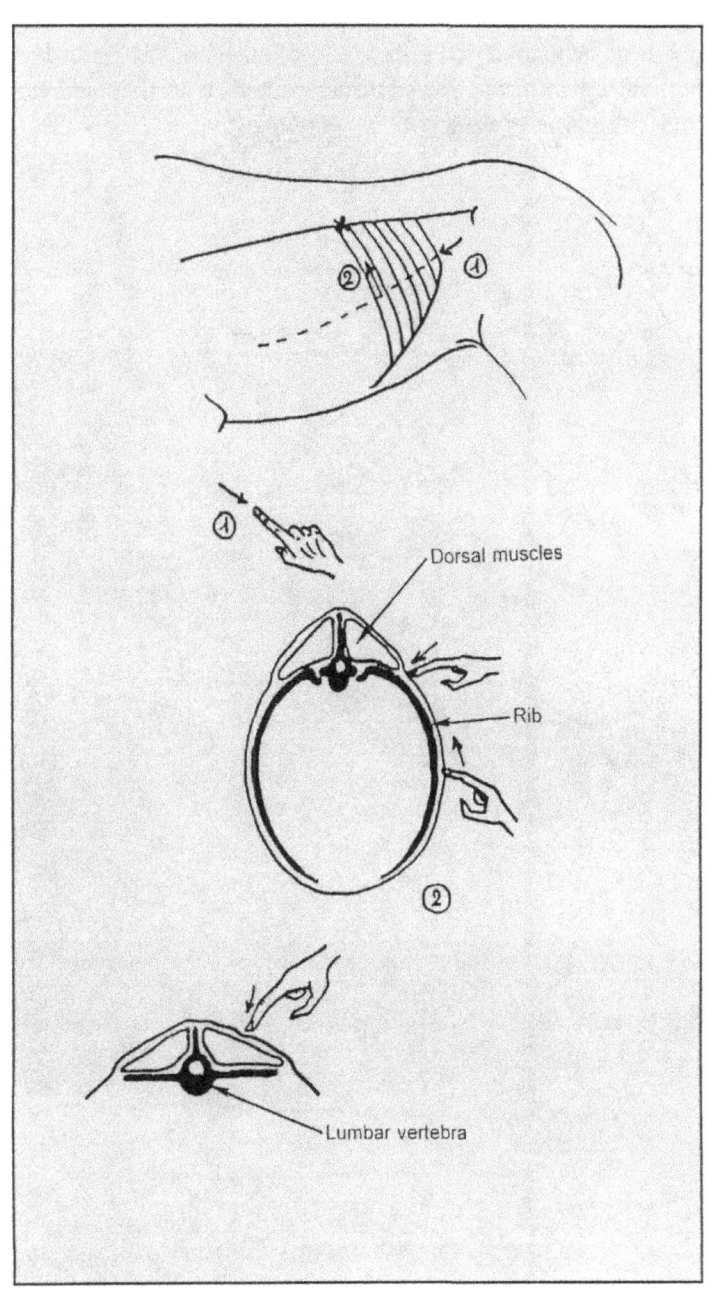

points go by symmetrical pairs and therefore have to be spotted on both sides of the horse. The first times, you may mark the points you find with a piece of chalk.

Chapter 5

EQUINE COLIC

There is almost always a misunderstanding between riders and nonriders when it comes to colic. This term bears a particular meaning with the horse.

Speaking of a human or a dog, when one speaks of colic, one evokes essentially a diarrhea, since with them it is the most frequent visible symptom associated with abdominal pain. But with a horse, it is most often the opposite. This apparent contradiction can be explained when one knows that colic means in fact "sharp pain in the large intestine."

For the equine, the word was extended to a whole set of abdominal pains due to diverse causes, but whose main symptoms are rather comparable. It therefore would be more proper to speak of a "colic syndrome," a syndrome being, by definition, a set of symptoms very often associated, but which can be associated as well in different afflictions. The best example of syndrome is fever: an abnormally high temperature is a symptom which does not have much of a meaning when it is isolated; it is by contrast an important symptom of the syndrome fever when it is accompanied with general exhaustion, cricks, acceleration of the pulse, etc.

An equine colic is therefore a set of signs frequently associated, but which cannot indicate by themselves the precise trouble, or which organ is concerned. Diagnosing the exact location of the pain must be done by the veterinarian after a complete exam including auscultation, checking of the pulse, rectal palpation and other investigations. These techniques allow one to set in evidence possible serious lesions and establish a prognosis, but they often do not help in determining the location where the original spasm occurred, or its cause. While waiting for the arrival of the practitioner, every person present gives their opinion, since each has already seen at least one case which seems perfectly identical.

In this respect, I want to mention a detail which risks disappointing persons who, as there sometimes are, give peremptory advice without knowing anything of veterinary medicine, and who easily criticize the veterinarian while coming up with bogus proofs. I want to speak of the supporters of urinary colic who cry victory if the horse starts urinating as soon as he is feeling better, as well as those who see a confirmation of the digestive origin when the return to normalcy is accompanied with some droppings. This is not a proof that any one of them was right. Let me tell you indeed that there are cases when the horse cannot urinate because his bowels ache too much, and others when he cannot defecate because that would compress too much an aching bladder. In the same respect, when colic ceases upon the mere action of a diuretic, this is not enough proof that the real cause of the colic was there; even an ovary pain may be stopped in this way. The pain becoming rapidly a vicious circle, the feeling of well-being provided by the mere fact of urinating may relax so much the tension of the nervous system that the original spasm benefits from this general relaxation. When a person is bellyaching, making that person laugh may sometimes help, as everybody knows. Don't accuse me of reducing the treatment of colic to the mere fact of "changing the ideas." On the contrary, I want to show that it is a far more complex problem that some hold, who too often pretend that they would have done better than the veterinarian.

Unless the veterinarian finds a serious lesion showing that the animal is in a very serious state (an irreparably damaged organ), or a less serious requiring a surgical intervention, it may seem surprising that each practitioner sets out to implement a standard treatment he is accustomed to. Moreover, the owner has usually started the injection before the arrival of the veterinarian whose protocol he knows.

The explanation is very simple and risks coming as a shocker: medicine does not know how to treat a colic at the stage when it is only a set of functional troubles!

If any practitioner has a preference for an antispasmodic, with as good results as his colleagues have with others, it is because all these products have about the same reaction: they momentarily "unplug" the autonomic fibers, rather blindly as for the direction of their imbalance. When their effect ceases, the colic starts again if the imbalance has remained blocked at the same stage; rather often on the other hand, the cessation of the pain has allowed a relaxation of all the tensions and the resumption of all the regular oscillations which constitute balance.

When I say that medicine does not know how to treat a colic at a functional stage (hence before there are lesions), I don't mean to say it is inefficient, but I observe that it is blind. It rarely knows where the spasm lies, it too often ignores the direction of the imbalance, and anyway the therapeutic protocol depends more on habit and experience than on the case itself.

When veterinarians meet in symposiums in order to exchange news about the treatment of colic, the lectures deal with the fight against the state of shock, the state of the art techniques of abdominal surgery or, on the other hand, with food hygiene or other means of prevention. Even if the theme of the symposium is "the treatment of colic," they can only speak of the ways to avoid it or repair its consequences.

If I have been so bent on perfecting and verifying a technique of treatment based on ideas of acupuncture, it is because this kind of medicine, on the contrary, works perfectly at the functional stage: it knows where to act and in which direction according to each case. No anti-spasmodic, even the most judiciously chosen, has ever shown me the rapidity of action which a well-applied session of acupuncture has.

With the help of the following pages, without having to call yourself an acupuncturist, you will be capable of checking numerous cases of colic before they have created lesions and furthermore you will be capable of pointing out more precisely the organ where the trouble lies.

A - Impaction colic

It is the most common (the equivalent of constipation for the human); it is accompanied with a food overload in the large intestine which loses its peristalsis. Palpating the rectum, the veterinarian can clearly feel a full, hard, and inert colon. The caecum itself, which is the big bacterial digestive tank before the colon, is often full and lifeless.

The arrest of the oscillations of the autonomic system in this case is due to an excess in the action of the sympathetic fibers. The action of these nerves slows down the contractions of the intestine, stops the secretion of the glands of the digestive track, and above all exaggerates the re-absorption of the liquids contained in the colon. This latter effect entails an abnormal dehydration of the food in the process of being digested, and it is all the more difficult for the intestine to help it going through.

You can verify yourself the stopping of the contractions of the caecum by applying the ear in the hollow part of the right flank of the horse. In the course of a normal digestion, one hears at this place a rather impressive contraction about every two minutes. It suffices to have listened to it once to remember it and recognize it easily.

With impaction colic, one observes a silence sometimes accompanied with "gargles" without detectable rhythm. If you hear in addition a kind of "little bells" ringing, the case is more serious; this noise corresponds to a bursting out of bubbles due to the exaggerated fermentation of the stagnating food.

In case of complete abdominal silence accompanied with numerous "little bells," and moreover if the animal is really exhausted, one should always think of the possibility of a real occlusion or the torsion of the small intestine, which obligatorily requires the veterinarian, and often the surgeon. This will not prevent you from intervening as he is on his way to you since some cases can yield in this way, and anyway your action will help the horse coping with the pain while waiting.

Impaction colic is found first with horses who have eaten too much straw, and those who are fed with pellets.

Although all the horses may be subject to it, you will notice that those who are "pigeon toed" are much more predisposed than the others to this kind of colic. The laws of traditional acupuncture, based on the circulation of the Energy in the meridians, explain very well this predisposition: a pigeon toed horse is a horse whose front feet horn grows faster on the inside front part of the hoof, which turns his feet inward.

The impaction colic is due to an excess of Energy in the meridian of the large intestine, and this meridian starts its course at the inside front part of the front hoof. The excessive growth of horn expresses clearly the excess of Energy of this meridian and points to the basic imbalance of these horses.

You will observe as well that those who are splay footed are more frequently afflicted with spasmodic colic or diarrheas. The same applies if one considers now the meridian of the small intestine or the meridian of "triple heater." The study of the connection between the weak points (and hence the basic pathology) of the animal and the shape of his feet allowed me to retrieve the disposition of these meridians with the horse; and the use of these meridians on this basis seems very satisfactory.

The traditional Chinese documents we have at hand enumerate many points and their indications, but do not indicate meridians with the animals.

If your horse is very pigeon toed, consider nourishing him the traditional way (i.e., no pellets. -*Translator*) and limiting somewhat his intake of straw. But let's not forget that fibers are still necessary to stimulate by irritation the contractions of his lazy intestine.

An impaction colic may sometimes last for several days in a row. The method indicated in this book may then suffice if you monitor some details: the animal must drink, he should be neither agitated nor exhausted, and above all you must check regularly your efficiency in the maintenance of the digestive transit. If you succeed in restarting it two or three times a day, the result will be good.

If, on the other hand, your action is less and less efficient, think of verifying whether the points indicated have changed, modifying your intervention accordingly, and quit insisting if the answer is not immediate. In such an acute case, it is wiser to have your veterinarian check regularly the progress of trouble. There is of course no contra-indication in continuing both treatments together if the veterinarian deems it appropriate.

In an impaction colic, the principal point which reacts to the tests of palpation, and must therefore be treated, is situated between the two last ribs. It is the Shu point of the meridian of the large intestine and, according to the technique described above, one finds it in the first intercostal interval one meets, on the edge of the common mass of the dorsal muscles (Fig. 4). The Chinese call it "Ta Shang Shu."

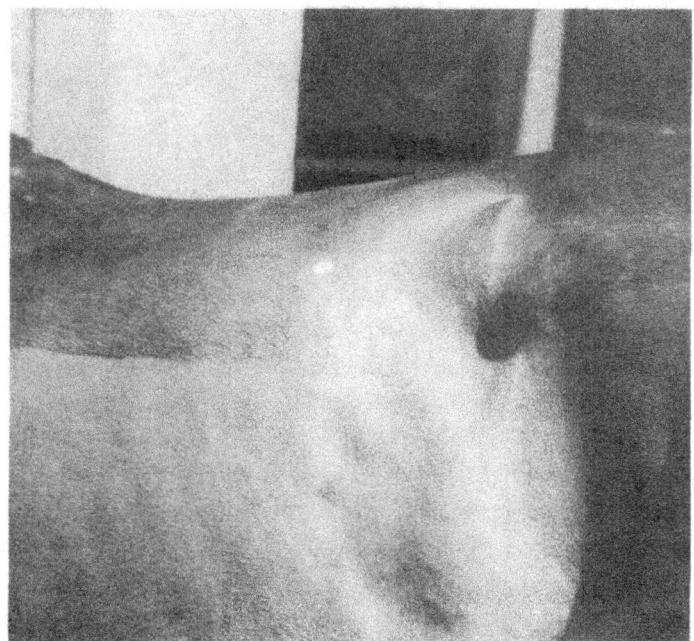

Fig. 4 - Ta Shang Shu

Often, with this very colic, you will also have found that the Shu point of the spleen ("Pi Shu") in the third intercostal space tested positively (Fig. 5); you will have treated it first, because it is always less unsettled and yields easily to massage.

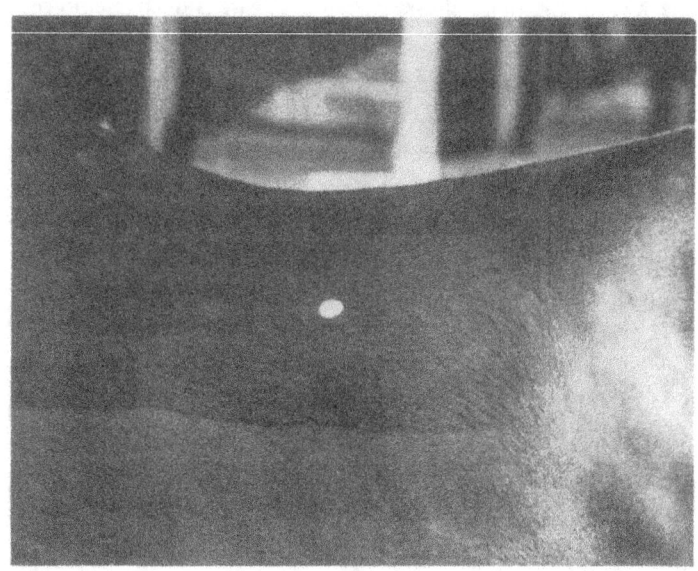

Fig. 5 - Pi Shu

If you do not forget that you must treat both sides of the horse, these two points (Ta Shang Shu and Pi Shu) will suffice, if the caecum is still not blocked. In the much more frequent case when the stasis (which is the stagnation of the digestive process) concerns also the caecum, you will have subsequently to massage a specific point for this organ. It is not a Shu point and it presents in addition the particularity of being unilateral. Like the caecum, it is situated on the right side of the animal and is to be found at mid-distance between the point of the hip and the eighteenth rib—the first to be found when counting them from rear to front (Fig. 6).

Don't hesitate massaging this point energetically for at least three

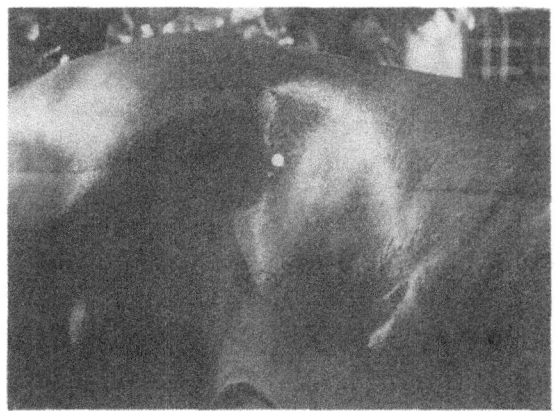

Fig. 6

to four minutes. This will restart the contractions of the caecum which you will hear clearly in the meantime as you will feel them under your finger.

For this point, you also can use a couch grass (stiff bristled) brush in this way: press and rotate in place without rubbing the skin, but as if you wanted to sink the bristles into the skin (Fig. 7).

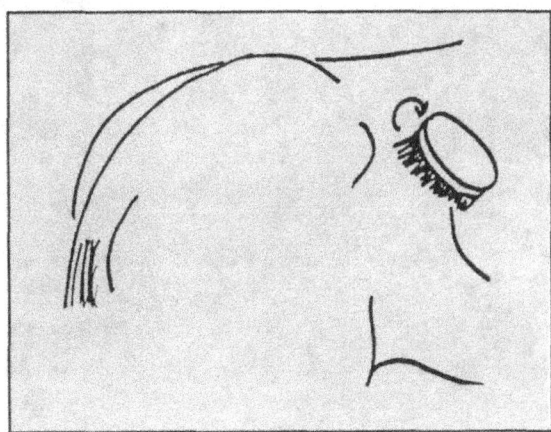

Fig. 7

A last important point, which you will find in diverse types of colic, works primarily on the abdominal pain. It is the swelling of the abdomen which makes it react, whatever its cause; most colic being accompanied with fermentations and therefore with a more or less important flatulence, it is not surprising that it is often indicated.

This point is bilateral, under the horse's belly. The horse feels it very well, since it is precisely the spot he bumps with his hind ankle. When you rub the horse's belly with a bundle of straw, it is on this point that you are working, and you will be more efficient if you know how to localize it.

It is called Yun Men and is situated about eight centimeters (three inches) off the medial line, right where the belly is at its lowest when one looks at the horse from profile (Fig. 8). Watch out, since the horse tends to kick with his ankle as soon as one strokes the point. It may be prudent to have someone take the front leg of the horse as you massage this point. If you prefer the friction with a bundle of straw, do it crosswise in order to treat both sides together.

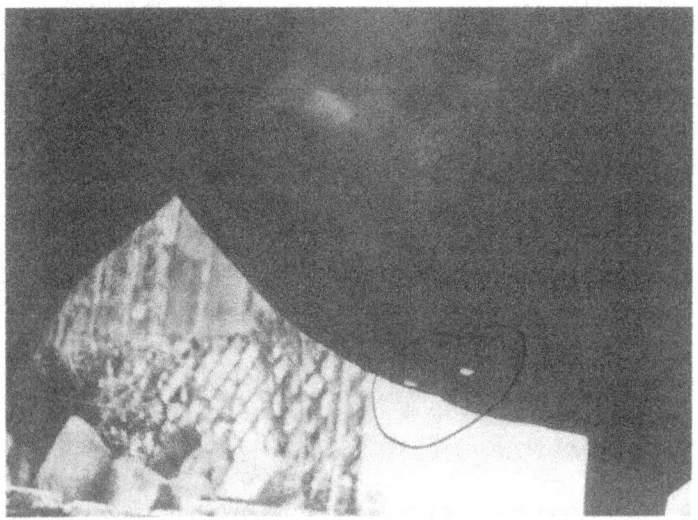

Fig. 8 - Yun Men

B - Acute gastric indigestion

The dilatation and inflammation of the stomach may, if they occur suddenly, entail cases of colic, sometimes worrying ones. The main cause is the rapid ingestion of a large volume of cold water or spoiled food. There are several known favoring factors, such as parasitism, anxiety and the gastritis which does not fail to accompany it, "wind sucking," etc.

Although the stomach alone is usually concerned, gastric colic is sometimes associated with another portion of the digestive tract.

The pain is visibly important, and some of the symptoms are characteristic enough to orient the investigation toward the stomach. More particularly, the horse breathes haltingly, he yawns noisily, "sucks in" his belly and looks as if he wanted to throw up, or he belches frequently.

The point allowing us to recognize a gastric colic is the Shu point of the stomach (Wei Shu) in the sixth intercostal space (Fig.9).

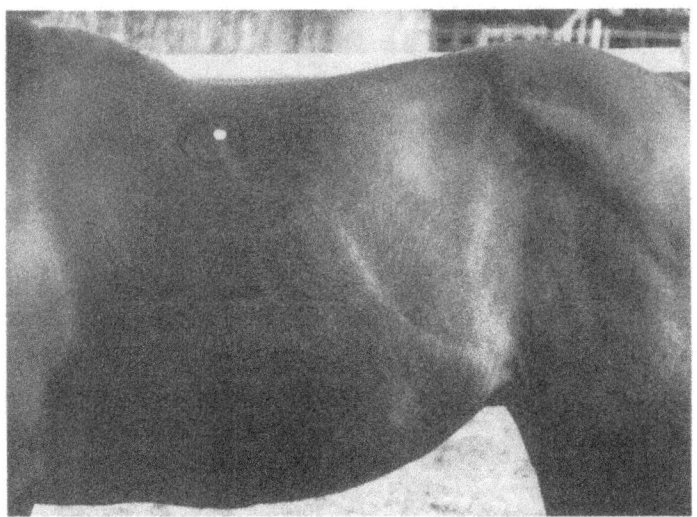

Fig. 9 - Wei Shu

If the symptoms are alarming, as it often happens, limit yourself to diagnosing, for this is an emergency. The veterinarian will relieve your horse much faster than you could have done, by emptying his stomach with a naso-esophageal probe. If this is not done rapidly, there are two serious risks which may place the horse in great danger:

- When a horse succeeds in vomiting, the particular conformation of his palate is such that the content of his stomach flows back into the nasal cavities and the inhalation which follows carries away the whole into the bronchial tubes. There can be choking, or at least infection and even gangrene of the lungs.
- Another anatomical oddity of the horse lies in the entry of his stomach which prevents some of them from vomiting.

The nausea is extremely painful and it may happen then that the stomach gets rent. The swollen stomach may also burst out if the horse lets himself fall violently because of the pain.

The rupture of the stomach, although it brings about an immediate relief which has deceived many a one, is irremediably lethal for the horse.

So do not try to treat this affection, but rather profit by your advantage to diagnose it rapidly, and call your veterinarian at once.

C - Spasmodic colic

The spasmodic colic is linked to an imbalance of the autonomic system which corresponds to a predominance of the action of the parasympathetic fibers.

Take note that I'm saying it is *linked*, I am not saying it is *inevitably* due to this imbalance; the latter is sometimes the consequence of another primary cause, but the healing cannot be obtained as long as it persists. It is my belief that in medicine, if one wants to broaden the span of the therapeutic possibilities, one has to be willing to quit the classical process of reasoning from cause to effect. Facing a set of symptoms, one is used to deciding "a priori" that one of them is the cause of such another, which is thence considered its effect, this latter being the cause for a third one, and so forth. This "scale wise" process is a kind of reasoning which may lead to an impasse.

If one is capable of imagining that the cause is perhaps only the consequence, or that both are sometimes mere consequences of a cause one has failed to see, or which perhaps does not exist, one will then have many more possibilities to treat a disease. It is sad to see patients condemned because a single and compartmented intellectual process did lead to an inescapable conclusion, above all when this process does not allow one to tackle the problem from another angle.

After this little digression, let's return to the spasmodic colic.

The parasympathetic nervous fibers are in charge of accelerating and increasing the secretion of the glands at the expense of the re-absorption of the liquids. This is therefore the reverse picture with respect to the colic of stasis.

Diarrhea is the first stage of such an imbalance, but with the horse, this imbalance is sometimes so rapid and so intense that it also leads to a stopping of the intestine; complex phenomena of anarchy in many diverse modes of contraction of the intestinal wall conflict with normal peristalsis and jam the whole transit.

While the impaction colic is comparable to a traffic jam on a highway during the rush hour, the spasmodic colic is the accident which happens in a moving traffic when cars move too fast.

With this type of colic, the main Shu points to consider are the Shu point of the small intestine (Hsiao Shang Shu) and that of the Triple Heater (San Shiao Shu).

The Shu point of the Triple Heater is situated on the same line as the points already described, in the fourth intercostal space you are going to feel (Fig. 10). You will find it much indicated in the cases when the horse is perspiring abnormally; it is a point of command of the parasympathetic system. I mention one more time that it is bilateral like practically all the others.

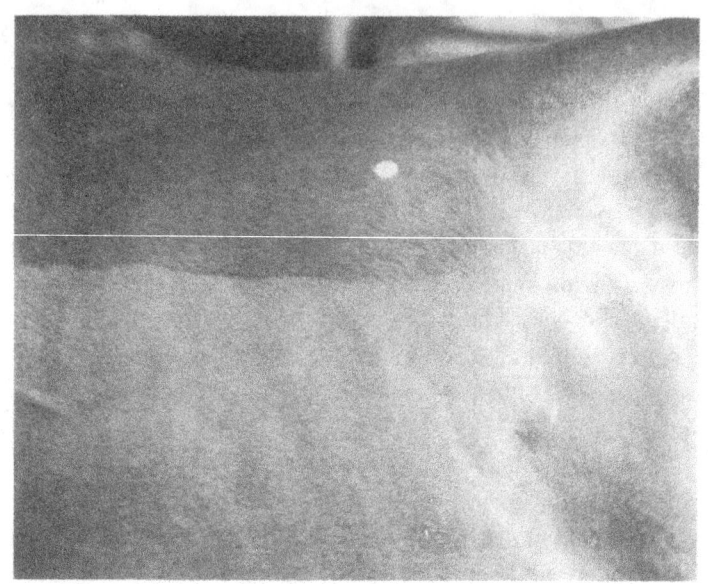

Fig. 10 - San Shiao Shu

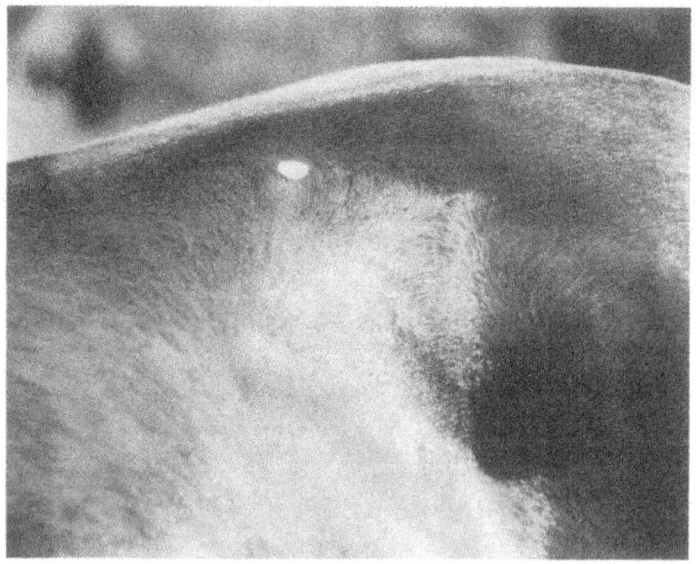

Fig. 11 - Shu point of small intestine

The Shu point of the small intestine is a little bit more difficult to localize: one finds it at the level of the lumbar vertebrae (the "loins" of the horse). It can be felt at mid-distance between the spinal column and the edge of the muscles of the common mass, two spaces back from the level of the last rib—between the second and third lumbar vertebrae (Fig. 11).

One can also find the Shu point of the spleen (Pi Shu, already mentioned), but it is less obvious, and therefore one should massage it and make it yield in the first place.

The Shu Men point (pain due to belly's distension) is generally indicated also in most cases of spasmodic colic.

The intussusception, or "invagination" of a segment of the intestine (the fact that a portion of the bowel turns inside out like a glove finger) is a form of spasmodic colic. It is a case when the anarchy of the contractions is such that a hyperactive portion of the intestine "engulfs" the more lifeless preceding portion, as when one turns the finger of a glove inside out.

If this process is started, your massage will have no effect whatsoever and surgery is very likely to be required. It will be the task of your veterinarian to diagnose and make a decision about what has to be done.

Real acupuncture, combined with rectal manipulations of the intestine, may overcome such cases if they are recent and if there are still no fibrinous adhesions, but this is another story.

I mentioned this because, knowing that it may happen, you will intervene all the sooner in the case of a spasmodic colic in order to regularize the transit before such a lesion appears.

D - Diarrhea

I have already mentioned that colic is a syndrome which involves pain as one of its main symptoms; therefore diarrhea does not always pertain to it. There are indeed numerous cases of chronic diarrhea which are absolutely painless and which therefore do not belong to

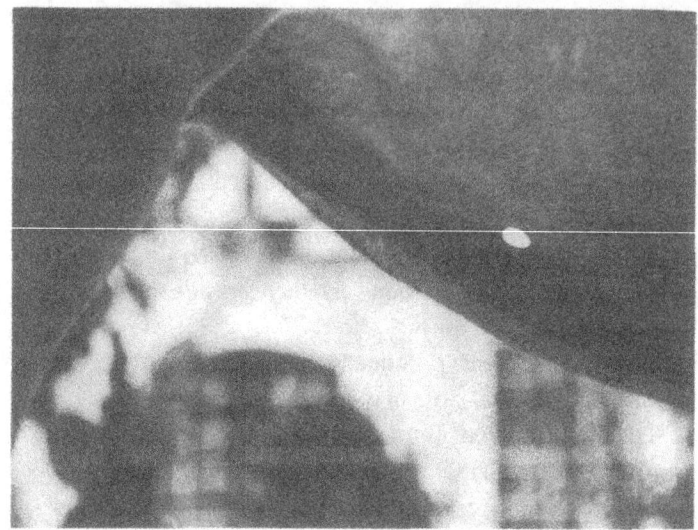

Fig. 12 - Tien Chu

the colic syndrome.

If I make a point to mention this right now, it is on the one hand because diarrhea, in its acute form, is very often a colic, and on the other hand because it is always treated like a spasmodic colic at the level of the Shu points. The only difference is that you will in addition treat a point specific to the diarrhea symptom, which is very efficient.

Before all, take notice that if the diarrhea is accompanied by a great pain, it is better not to waste time before calling the veterinarian. If the animal is very agitated, tries to lie down but doesn't do it, if he breathes noisily and shivers, when he emits jets of liquid matter, always think of a possible acute crisis of melioidosis or piroplasmosis. These diseases are particularly serious and require a rapid application of a specific treatment by your veterinarian.

In the case when it is not about one of those two diseases, you will anyway need him in order to re-hydrate your horse and make up for the enormous loss in liquids which weakens him and sets him all the more in peril. Never forget that an organism with diminished Energy reserves reacts less well to acupuncture.

The point for diarrhea (Tien Chu) is very easy to locate since it is under the belly, roughly between the umbilicus and the stifle, precisely on the circular "cow lick" one can see on this spot (Fig. 12).

A brush used as for the point of the caecum will allow one to treat it easily, as well as a fairly energetic friction with a bundle of straw (this on both sides of the horse, of course).

In the presence of a horse afflicted with a chronic diarrhea without colic, you will treat only this point, but you will repeat your intervention daily for about two minutes on each side. Fairly often, this is enough to bring the droppings to normalcy, at least as long as you compel yourself to do the task. If the response is positive, try and interrupt the treatment from time to time to see if the result lasts.

E - Urinary colic

With this chapter, we have at last the occasion to expose those I have already spoken of, who have precisely seen the same colic happen, and know at once, definitely, whether it is about a urinary or digestive problem.

You will have the last word, since there is a Shu point which answers only in case of urinary colic. This point is situated at about eight centimeters (three inches) on both sides of the median line of the back, at the level between the last lumbar vertebra and the sacrum. To find and test it, you will follow the back's median line, on top of the lumbar spines, and you will spot the lumbo-sacral space where your finger sinks, before the pelvis. The point is situated on both sides of this depression (Fig. 13).

On the rare charts the Chinese have transmitted to us, this point is called Shen Shu, which means "the command point of the meridian of the kidneys." I personally prefer to call it the urinary point, since it commands the pathways of urinary evacuation; the real point for the kidneys being situated at the level of the space between the two first lumbar vertebrae. For the human, this Shen Shu point bears

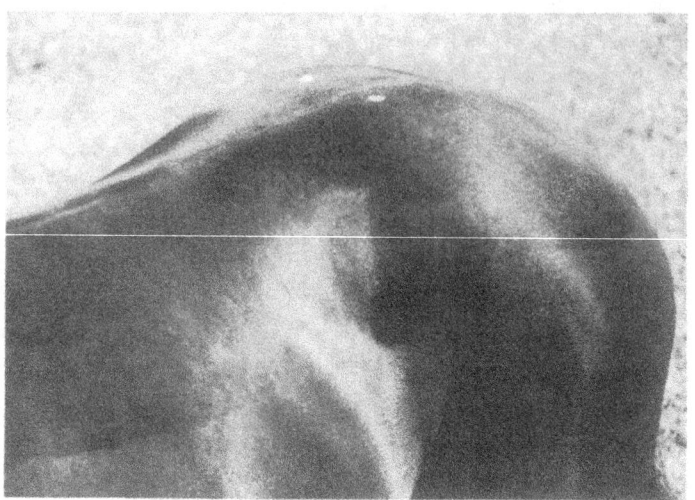

Fig. 13 - Prang Kwan Shu

the name of Prang Kwan Shu.

Its indication and action would rather correspond to those of the Prang Kwan Shu of human charts (urinary retention and pain accompanying micturition).

Urinary colic is due to a reflex spasm of the urinary duct (ureter). This reflex may be linked to an inflammation of microbian as well as non-microbian origin, or to the presence of stones in the ureter.

One can easily treat this point on both sides simultaneously with only one hand. The horse parks out almost immediately, and seems to labor. In the end, he relieves himself by urinating. Keep on massaging as he is in the process of urinating, since he would quit at once if you stopped your action.

At this point I would like to mention, and this is perhaps the more useful, that this point is very convenient in the case of a horse's refusing to urinate in a trailer. It is obviously less dangerous to relieve him in this way than to disembark him on an expressway, and he will be in a better shape for the show he is heading to!

Note that you won't have any result if the bladder is empty.

Chapter 6

OVARY PROBLEMS

This chapter forms a transition between the chapter about colic and the following, since we will speak of diverse gynecological problems, but first and foremost of the types of "colic" which may accompany some ovary problems.

Ovaries are endocrine glands and are therefore under the control of the pituitary gland, itself narrowly connected to the nervous system. The psyche may play a part (cause or consequence...). I have known a mare whose ovarian colic, which would regularly and systematically precede her being in seasons, would yield to an intravenous injection done with an empty syringe. Nothing was injected, but this act was nevertheless necessary to trigger off normal and painless heats!

Whether it is about a fortuitous ovary colic on occasion of a laborious ovulation, or about practically constant pains linked to a chronic inflammation of the ovaries, the point to work will always be the same; it offers particularities which are worth elaborating further.

This point is not featured on the Chinese charts we have at hand. These latter indicate a somewhat neighboring point which is clearly less efficient. Whereas the Chinese point is on the edge of the common mass (like the others) just behind the last rib, the point I am proposing to you lies a few centimeters lower, against this very rib. If you follow the back edge of this rib going downwards, you will find this point in an indentation, just before the curve which links the rib to the cartilaginous costal arch (Fig. 14).

A particularity of this point is that its reaction is perfectly lateral:

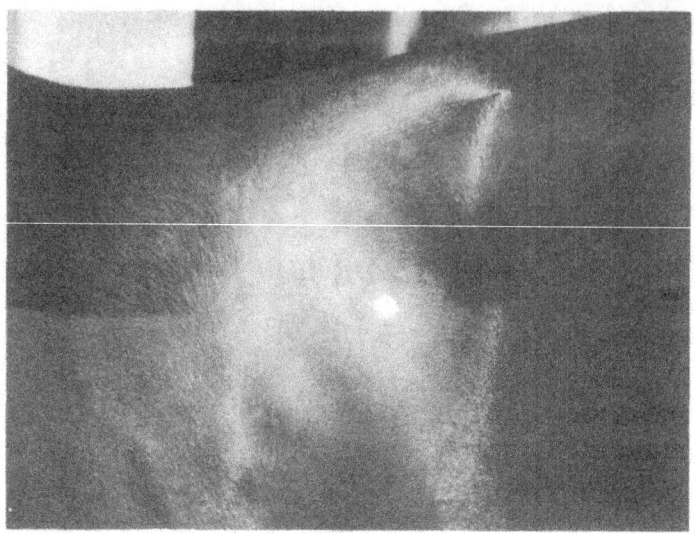

Fig. 14 - "Ovary" point

it answers indeed only on the side of the afflicted ovary.

When buying a mare, you will know thanks to this point if she has healthy ovaries without having to resort to palpation. I have never observed ovary perturbations with a mare without a positive answer from this point on one side at least. It gives information on the good functioning of the ovary and reacts irrespective of the direction of imbalance. It gives sometimes better information than would palpation of the ovaries, for instance when it reacts in the case of ovaries which, although appearing normal when palpated, are blocked from a hormonal point of view (and it then allows one to restore their functioning!).

I have been able to assess the great interest of this point in the domain of breeding as well as riding. Its stimulation triggers off the ovulation when it is ready to come about. It is moreover amusing to observe that when a stallion sidles a mare in heat, he begins by nipping precisely this point! This is not the only example of instinctive utilization of an acupuncture point by an animal; humans as well resort to it unconsciously in some situations.[1] I shall come back to it later on.

Massaging this point for one or two minutes on both sides the day a mare is to be bred, increases the chances of fecundation and brings a difficult mare to lend herself more freely to the protocol which awaits her at the stud farm!

In the field of riding, you certainly know about mares who, although normal the rest of the time, are difficult to work from the end of November on, and sometimes until March. The explanation is simple: it is a known fact that, in our hemisphere, there are real ovulations with the mare only from December to July. Fairly often the hormone level necessary for the ovulation is too low at the beginning of the season. The follicle formed in the ovary does not come to maturity and therefore does not split open; it remains for some time in the shape of a cyst which recedes little by little and impairs by its presence the following ovulation(s). This circumstance reflects on the behavior and performances of the mare, through the hormonal imbalance as well as mechanically through the pain induced in the affected ovary.

If your mare becomes nervous around the first of December, brush the caudal (back) edge of the last rib, on both sides, two or three days in a row, right before working. The first ovulation will be thorough and the normal cycle will be set for the rest of the season.

This technique is very efficient, and I know mares who require this specific treatment at the same time every year and then go on without problems.

The hormonal deficiency observed on the occasion of these troubles is probably due to too much time spent in a stall. The organism is not submitted to the periodic variations of solar light, and the stimulation of the pituitary gland is then anarchic (the pituitary gland is an organ which acts as a relay between the nervous system and the hormonal system).

The frequent failures in classical treatments of these troubles can be explained by the fact that the pituitary gland "understands" still less what's going on when a hormone is injected without its (the pituitary's) having had the time to ask it from the ovaries. It may even happen that confronted by the massive delivery of an unexpected hormone, the pituitary panics, and then "clams up" and forgoes any further intervention in this domain.

This explanation is mine, but it shows clearly how the classical therapy may sometimes be responsible for serious troubles with a mare and possibly call into question her future as a brood mare.

By treating the first troubles the way I am proposing, you not only will be more rapidly efficient, but you won't jeopardize your hopes as a breeder as well.

The same problem happens for more serious ovarian troubles, but then one has to resort to real acupuncture with its theories on Energy in order to restore harmony; the limited information given here does not suffice.

If the ovarian pain is very important, you may in addition massage another point right before working. This point will be particularly useful in case of an ovarian "colic." The Chinese call it "San Yin Tsiao."

You will treat it with a brush, holding the rear hoof as if you were cleaning it. To avoid the regrettable consequences of an always possible reaction from the mare, position yourself to the right for the left hind leg, and vice-versa. This point is much used in human acupuncture and, for the mare, is situated inside the leg, against the big vein (internal saphenous), at the spot where it bifurcates perpendicularly forward (Fig. 15). Hold the foot with one hand and with the other hand, brush the internal face of the leg for twenty to thirty seconds, while pressing moderately.

Every woman should learn how to recognize this point on themselves since it is very efficient against periodic as well as ovarian pains. It is located a hand width above the ankle, against the rear edge of the tibia. But it would be ill advised to use the same brush as for a horse! (It is the point I mentioned in the lines above, the one which is concerned when one "plays footsie.")

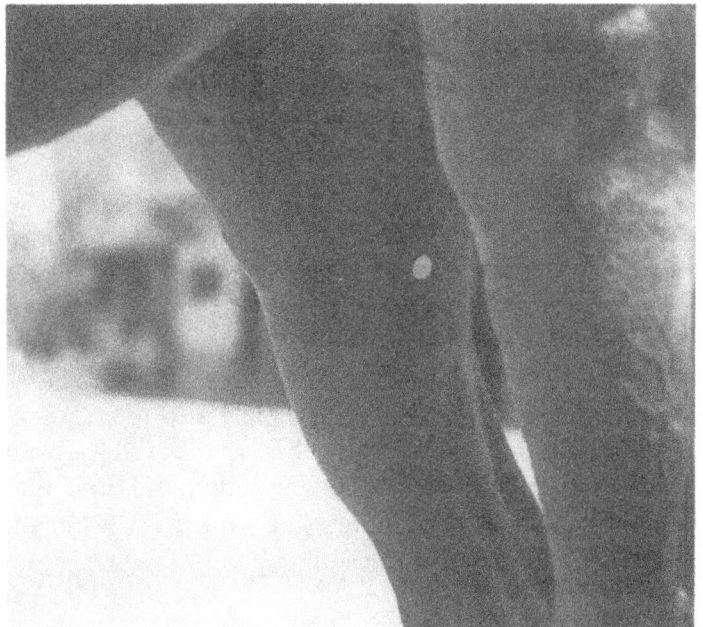
Fig. 15 - San Yin Tsiao

Let's come back to the point "of the ovaries," behind the last rib, and speak of its utility with the male and with the gelding.

The nervous sympathetic pathways for the testicles and their envelopes (scrotal sacs) are the same as those of the ovaries. All these organs indeed have the same embryological origin, and it is only during their growth that they migrate toward different positions, all the while keeping their original connections. One realizes therefore the efficacy of this point for an inflammation of the testicles (orchitis) and in the case of pains provoked by a too short or retracted cord. This point relaxes the muscle of the scrotal sacs (cremaster) and, by relaxing it, facilitates the descent of the corresponding testicle.

With a gelding hampered by the adhesion of this muscle to the scar of castration, this won't loosen the scar tissue, but will momentarily relax the contraction of the cremaster, and you will be better off using your horse in the following hour.

When a gelding you don't know offers the same answer for the testing of this point as would a mare with ovarian problems, you can practically affirm that he is hampered by scars resulting from his castration.

The same positive test with a stallion allows one to be certain that one of his testicles is ill descended, or that he underwent at one time a big inflammation (orchitis, or twisting, for instance).

Beware, however, of not tinkering with this point with a stallion afflicted with a strangled unguinal hernia, since albeit the point reacts in this case as well, its stimulation would have no effect at all. A horse's strangled unguinal hernia can only be treated surgically, and one knows that the intervention must be done within six hours, to stand any chances for success. Real acupuncture, combined with transrectal manipulations of the intestine may succeed, but it is a dangerous game, since time is limited!

---

[1] Asthmatic people, when they feel an attack coming, massage their sternum with their fingers, right where it presents an indentation: it is about the Tran Chong point, which is a very efficient way of fighting bronchial spasms.

Several other points mentioned in this book are used instinctively in this way: when pondering on some matter, one reaches a better concentration by pinching the base of the nose, between the eyebrows, on the In Tran point.

Everybodie knows the expression "playing footsie." If one does this on the inside part of the leg, right above the ankle, it is on a point which relaxes the neck of the womb and the vagina in the woman... I mention this for the record but there are numerous and more serious examples of the same which would be too long to develop here. Simply know that when you scratch a place of your body that itches suddenly, it is practically always related to a small imbalance of the organ corresponding to the meridian which passes through this spot.

Chapter 7

FOALING

Don't expect, thanks to elementary acupuncture, to unfold the leg of a foal that comes tucked up, or to straighten up the foal if it comes upside down. But on the other hand, you are going to be able to calm the mare, regularize her contractions, help in dilating the neck of her uterus, and finally facilitate the coming in of the milk if necessary.

To calm a mare made nervous by the foaling, you will use a point which works very well in all forms of anxiety. Everybody knows it, because one uses it instinctively to relax oneself by massaging one's eyebrows from the base of the nose toward the temples. The point is called In Tran and is situated, with the horse also, between the eyes, at mid-distance, on the top line of the orbit bones (Fig. 16).

Face your horse, set both hands on each side of the orbit bones, then press with both thumbs on the middle point and bring them progressively nearer the other fingers; repeat it, time and again.

One should take great care interrupting the contact when replacing the thumbs in the middle, because a massage toward the center would have the reverse effect, i.e., draw the attention and concentrate the mind on the ongoing problem. We all do this gesture when we ponder about a preoccupying subject and do not want our attention to be distracted.

Some remember that this point was used in the past, through repeated and regular soft tapping, to calm a horse during shoeing, or when giving a shot. One can help quite a bit a mare in this way during foaling, as we all know the disturbing role of anxiety in this occurrence. Before contemplating more or less complex and dangerous hormonal injections, you should know that many a time apparently impossible foaling will develop harmoniously through the mere effect of a minute dose of a sedative: yet it is surprising that so many obviously competent people ignore this.

Your action, as efficient as a sedative and devoid of risks, will allow you to avoid resorting to a sometimes necessary but never insignificant therapeutic arsenal.

To regularize the contractions of a laborious foaling, there is a possibility which doesn't concern the genital system or the nervous system. The contractions of the abdomen and the uterus use the diaphragm as a fulcrum and solicit it so much that it often ends up blocked, entailing a pain which impairs the regular execution of the whole process.

You will easily remove this obstacle by using the Shu point of the diaphragm (Ko Shu) which is located on the same line as the other Shu points, in the eighth intercostal interval—as always counting from rear to front (Fig. 17).

As with all the other points I mentioned, it reacts to the test only if it is indicated and massaging it rapidly results in a general relaxation with resumption of the contractions if their interruption was indeed due to this diaphragmatic problem.

When the mare is calm with regular contractions, and yet nothing is coming on, what then comes to mind is that we are dealing with a lack of dilation of the neck of the uterus, and often rightfully so. However, it may also be an ill positioning of the foal, to be taken care of by a veterinarian, whose work you will have facilitated anyway while waiting. But if the foal has come with both front legs forward, its nose set down onto them, and there is no further progression, do not hesitate to test the following point, and massage it if it reacts.

It is the Prang Kwan Shu I've spoken of, dealing with the urinary colic, since it is linked as much to the neck of the uterus as to the neck of the bladder. The same as it allows one to help urinate a horse who retains his urine, it contributes greatly in relaxing the neck of

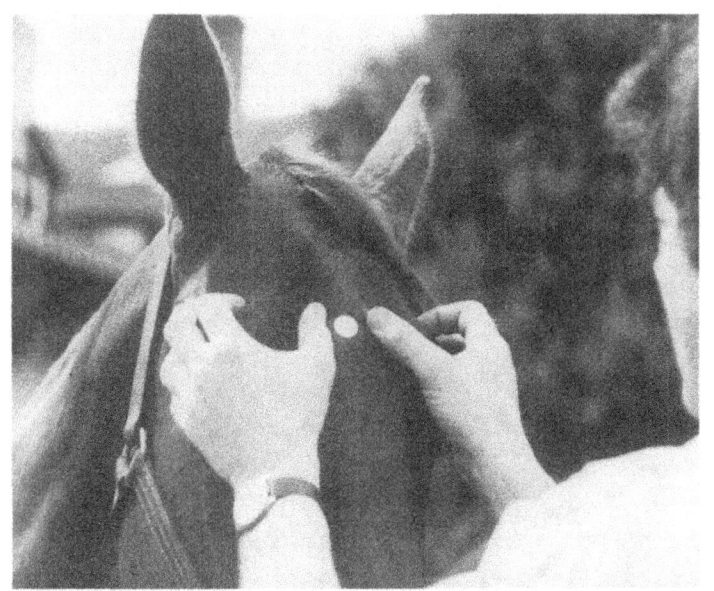

Fig. 16

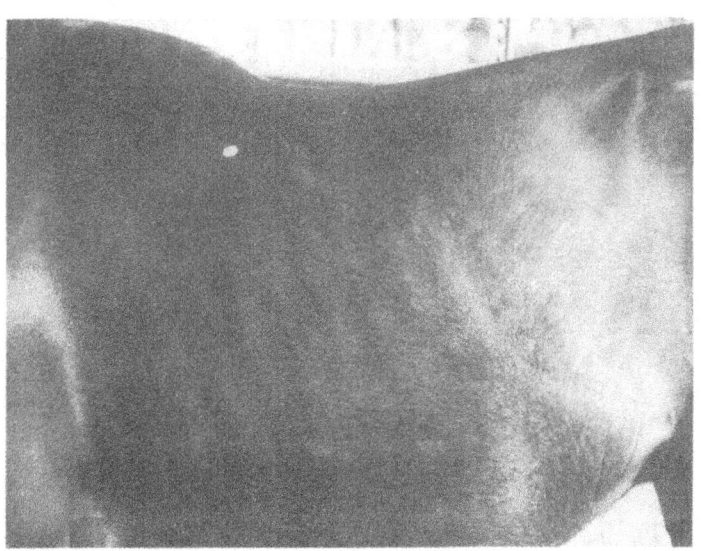

Fig. 17 - Ko Shu

the uterus with a mare in the process of foaling. I would like to remind the reader that it can be found on both sides of the space situated between the last lumbar vertebra and the sacrum (refer to Fig. 13).

Upon completion of the foaling, one may sometimes come across another problem, namely that of a mare whose milk does not come up, which may be due to two opposite phenomena.

Most often, the coming on of the milk is such that the subsequent congestion of the udders creates a pain which prevents the contraction of the ducts, hence the delivery of the milk, from happening. The mare therefore is upset by the attempts of the foal at sucking.

In traditional acupuncture, this event is linked to an abnormal excess of Energy in the meridian of the stomach. The udders are indeed situated on the course of this meridian, and it is the flow of Energy in its pathway which induces their activity. Another well known aspect of this phenomenon is that pregnant women experience nausea and stomach aches during the period when their breasts swell in preparation for their future work. For traditional acupuncture, lactation is a visible overflowing of the excess of Energy contained in the meridian of the stomach!

With the mare, it is frequent that the inflow of Energy is too brusque and cannot find an outlet; therefore you will have to abate the Energy ratio in the meridian. The point of "dispersion" of the meridian of the stomach is called Li Toe and is located on the cranial (front) part of the coronet of the hind hooves (above the toe, Fig. 18). Rub it with a finger, or a brush.

This point is also used for the mares who, although not pregnant, present an edema of the udders without any visible reason.

Conversely, there are foalings where the mare displays a markedly insufficient coming up of milk. The same type of reasoning explains why one can act in this case by massaging the point of stimulation of the stomach meridian. This latter lies on the cranial face of the crease of the hock, up against the tendon of the long digital extensor muscle. It is called Tsi Tsrie (Fig. 19). Don't use a brush on this spot, unless using it vertically (upright). Treat it several times a day, and

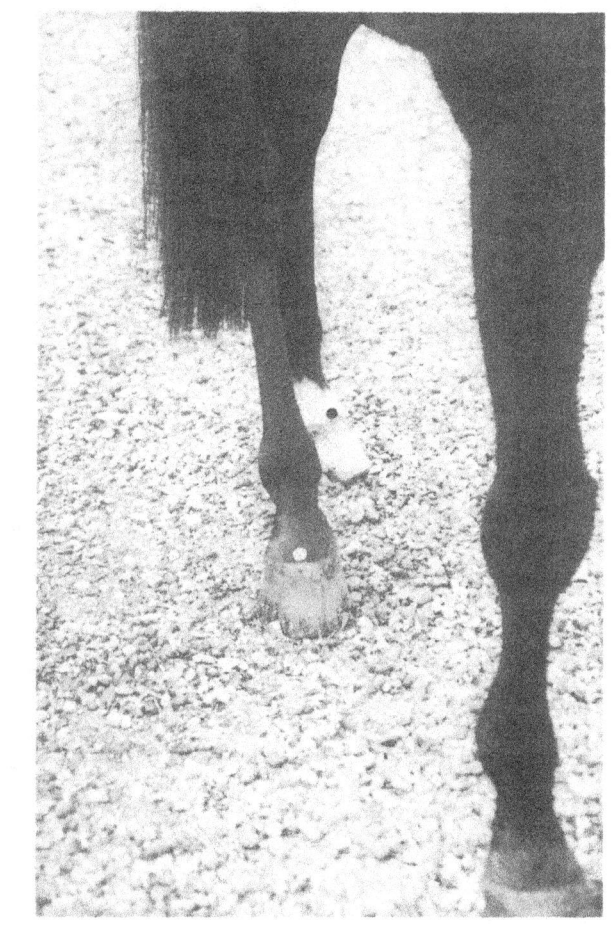

Fig. 18 - Li Toe

you will thus maintain the lactation. (An injection of water, with a "Dermo-jet,"™ on this point on each hock may suffice to bring about spectacular results.)

Now that birth has taken place, let's focus on the foal and see first how we can help, in addition to the usual procedures, if breathing is slow in coming about.

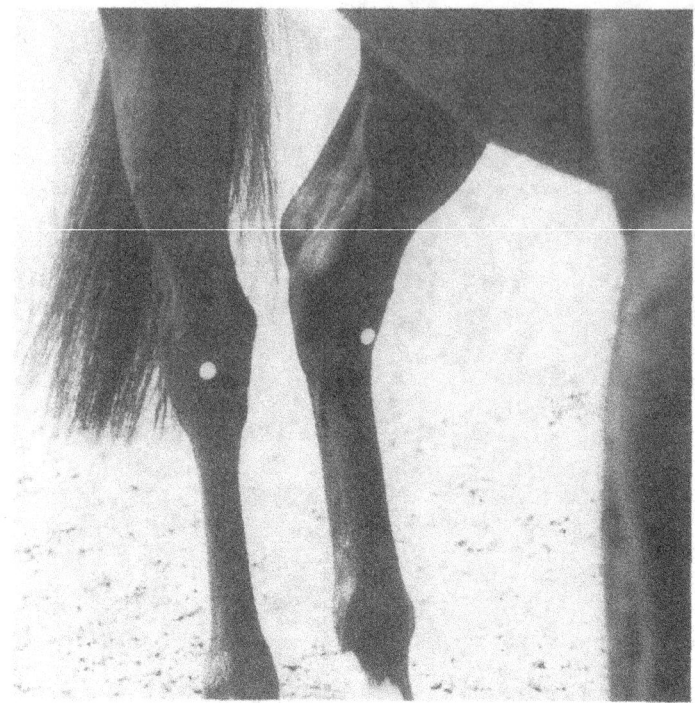

Fig. 19 - Tsi Tsrie

Two points are efficient in this case, but one must know how to differentiate their indications: each of them stimulates the respiration, but one of them starts an inhalation whereas the other induces, on the contrary, an exhalation.

The first, Ren Chong, is situated on the tip of the nose, on the median line. In fact, it is even in the thick of the upper lip, two thirds of the distance between the edge of the lip and its attachment to the gum, exactly where the membrane starts which links the upper lip to the gum (Fig. 20). Take the lip at this point between thumb and index finger, and squeeze strongly, if necessary by pulsations. With the other hand, try to keep the tongue stuck out to help the air come in. This point is the more efficient of the two, but it offers a formal

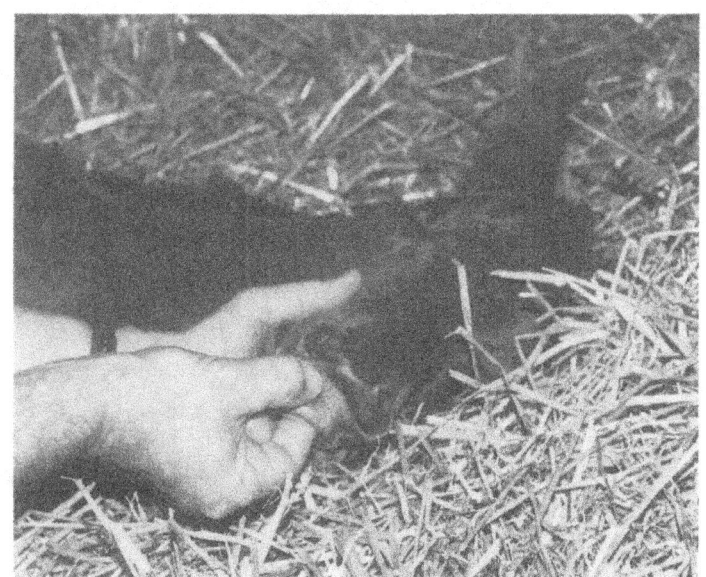

Fig. 20 - Ren Chong

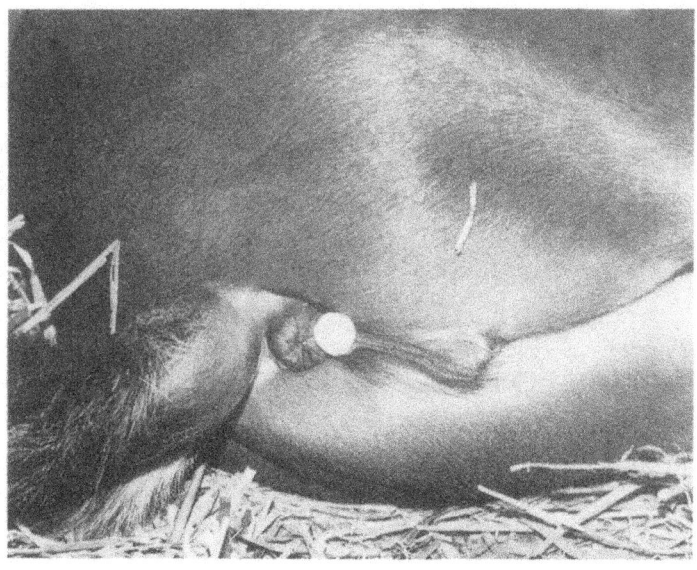

Fig. 21 - Roe Yin

contraindication: in the event of a foal who started breathing too soon and whose bronchi are encumbered with liquid, the strong inhalation it provokes would entail an invasion of the lungs by this liquid. Therefore this point should be reserved for the cases of real apnea, when the foal has not begun trying to breathe before getting out of the envelope.

For the other case, which is more of a suffocation than an apnea, one will be better off using the second point, which is at the other extremity. It is called Roe Yin and is located below the anus, at mid-distance between the anus and the vulva with the fillies (Fig. 21). One should never sting it or make any injection in this location with the male, since the penis extends exactly under it. Content yourself, as usual, with pressing on it while massaging the subcutaneous tissues. This point is less efficient and will work only if the lungs have been filled at least once. If the foal starts anyway by an inhalation, it means that the lungs were empty and that breathing has started on its own or thanks to whichever stimuli. The fact remains that this point will foster an exhalation if it is needed.

All is well now, the foal is breathing freely. But one may at this moment meet another problem: there are "clogged" foals which do not eliminate their meconium.

Do not try to make a foal suck by force, if it is in this situation, since it cannot have the reflex of suction as long as it is not freed from this problem. For it to get the instinctive urge to fill up its stomach, its whole digestive tube has to set to work and its contractions must be assured, which translates immediately through the ejection of the meconium. It is as if the room so created by the triggering off of the digestive transit was inducing the foal into filling it up through the other extremity.

All the breeders know that an enema will answer the question, but they also know, sometimes at their own expense, that it is a very delicate procedure, because of the extreme fragility of the rectal mucous with the newborn.

Besides, one knows that it is useful to massage the foal's belly and

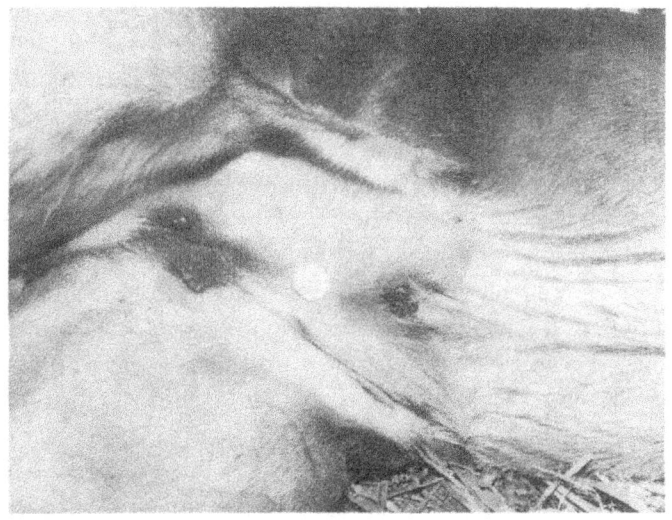

Fig. 22 - Kwan Yuan

I therefore would urge you to be more sophisticated. The exact point to be massaged is on the belly's median line, about mid-distance between the umbilical and the pubis (right before the sheath with the males). Rather than really massaging it, you will be more efficient by pressing your finger on it, with very little rotation; it is the pressure on the point which acts, essentially. This point is called Kwan Yuan (Fig. 22).

Take care, however, not to press thoughtlessly: the umbilical ring is close to it, and it is rather fragile.

We have here one more example of an instinctive gesture linked to acupuncture: this point is, as it happens, in the area where the mare licks her foal the most. Perhaps she is attracted by the umbilical cord, but the purpose is met.

Now that everything seems to be in order for the foal, let us come back to the mare, since there remains one more concern: the release of the placenta.

The organism of the mare is sometimes too tired to carry out the task, entailing some delay in the delivery of the placenta. One more time, this is a matter of spasm, but unlike in the cases we have heretofore examined, here we are dealing with a spasm which should come about, and fails to do so!

Normally, there should be at this moment an intense contraction from a multitude of small muscles in the wall of the womb. The purpose of this phenomenon is to block locally the blood circulation in order to disengage the placenta from the mucous membrane. Those two organs are narrowly intertwined during the pregnancy, somewhat like a "velcro" attachment; each micro-cavity of the uterine wall must then contract itself in order to push away the corresponding granule in the placenta.

The nerves of the autonomic system which have to send the order stem from the spinal cord at the level of the sacrum, and it is at the point of their emerging from it that you will have to work, if necessary.

This incident is due principally to the fact that the displacement of the sacrum necessary to the delivery of the foal may entail a momentary paralysis of the nerves I mentioned. A minor infection of the placenta adds to the problem of non-delivery, but it remains that the contraction is insufficient to overcome it.

Six points have to be stimulated together; they correspond anatomically to the "sacral holes" and their action is undeniable. They are located on top of the croup, on two longitudinal lines which converge toward the base of the tail (Fig. 23). By rubbing with a brush the two lines on both sides of the sacrum, you will feel the placenta become progressively heavier and finally fall within five to ten minutes.

Do not pull on the placenta as long as it does not come away, since the contraction is insufficient and there would be risk of hemorrhage if you pulled it off.

If you do not get any result within a short time, wait for fifty minutes before starting again: one should give the muscles of the uterine wall time to re-oxygenate, since your massage has blocked the microcirculation, which is all right but should not last.

These points, combined with that which relaxes the neck of the womb, help noticeably for the problems of discharges or neuritises which may accompany the foaling in the following days. Some day, we will see that real acupuncture solves these problems very well by itself, but we are not dealing with it presently. One should only think of verifying if the sacrum came correctly into its normal place and has not remained blocked in a twisted position because, potentially, this would impair the innervation and therefore the blood circulation in the whole genital area; and the blocking would then have to be released.

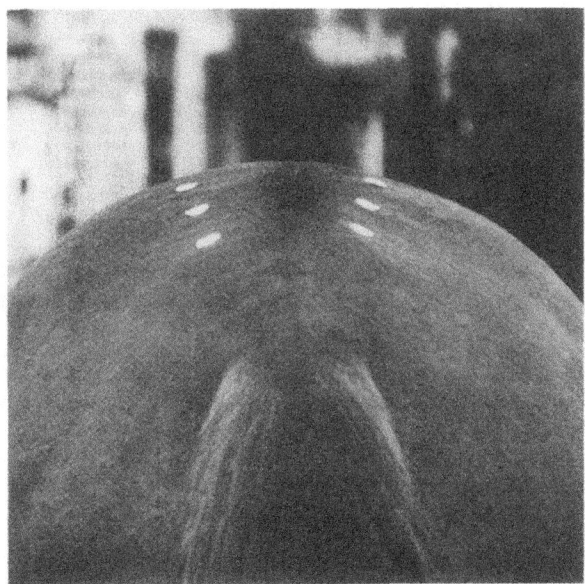

Fig. 23 - "Sacral holes" points

Chapter 8

CHRONIC PULMONARY EMPHYSEMA

Don't expect that you are going to heal your old "wheezing" horse. If it were possible, it would be everybody's knowledge! Nevertheless, you will be able to help him putting up better with his crises, and for some, you will even succeed in avoiding the onset of these so spectacular and disturbing crises that we would like to see gone forever!

You should know first that one of the classical treatments of emphysema based on time released corticoids is particularly dangerous and anyway is not a treatment in spite of the appearances.

If the emphysematous horse displays shortness of breath, it is because numerous alveoli in his lungs are destroyed and have lost their elasticity. The dilation of the lungs when they inhale then becomes painful, inducing the horse to limiting the amplitude of his breath, which helps in safeguarding the healthy parts, whose range of elasticity would be fully overcome by an unrestrained respiration. The only effect of the corticoids is to get rid of the pain in the stretched alveoli by suppressing the inflammation. Under the influence of such products, the horse does not feel any more that his lungs are fragile and he breathes joyfully, destroying them unknowingly at the same time. Five or six weeks later, when the effect of the drug is over, the horse is in a worse state than before, since one has only suppressed an "alarm bell."

Unless the purpose is to help an old retired horse enjoy the days he has left, one should not hesitate refusing such a "treatment" for a horse that is still being used.

I am not ruling out cortisone; it may turn out to be very useful for lungs which are the setting of an excessive microbian infection when it is necessary to limit the inflammation while the antibiotics are at work.

This digression was necessary; I have seen too many emphysematous horses "finished off" by corticoids. Yet their owners had been momentarily delighted by the results of such a fast and thorough working medication. One simply had forgotten to tell them that things would get eventually worse, and that this would be due to the medication.

What I am proposing is not to regenerate the fibrous alveoli or increase the elasticity of the healthy ones. Yet, it will allow the lessening of the spastic reaction of the bronchi which appears systematically on occasion of these fits.

First, the points acting directly on the lungs and their autonomic innervations are at your disposal. In fact, here again, the occurring spasm is linked to an imbalance of the sympathetic nervous system.

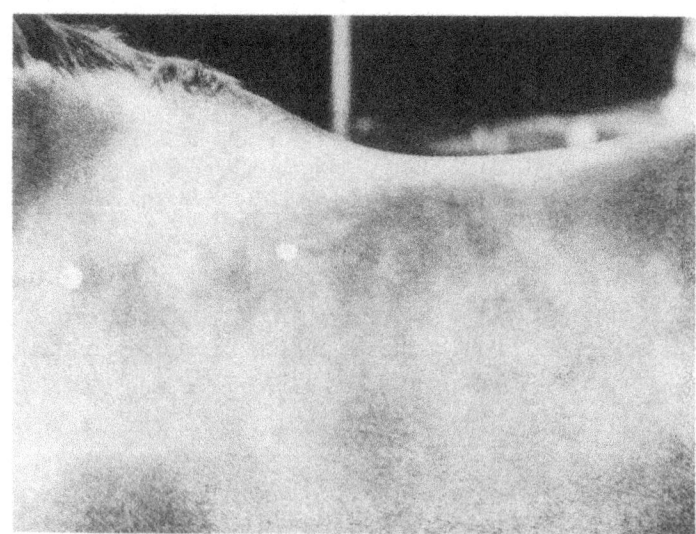

Fig. 24 - Fei Shu and Fei Shu Two

The Shu point of the lungs has two settings with the horse; it can be found in the ninth and thirteenth intercostal spaces (Fig. 24). The latter cannot be used with our method because of the presence of the shoulder muscles. The former—this of the ninth space—is fairly efficient with some horses, but because it's relatively difficult to reach I prefer another point which, although very far from the vertebral column, has a direct action on the autonomic system. It is located on the sternum and corresponds to an important nervous plexus.

All asthmatics know that this point hurts when they have a bout, even without touching it: all massage it instinctively and this gives them a relief. It is called Tran Chong and can be found with all the species where there is a "dip" in the sternum (Fig. 25). The feeling of well-being it provides comes fairly soon, but its massage should be soft, because it is particularly sensitive when it is indicated.

With many individuals, there is another possibility to check an acute crisis of emphysema. Although it may look surprising, one applies then to a meridian we already mentioned, that of the stomach!

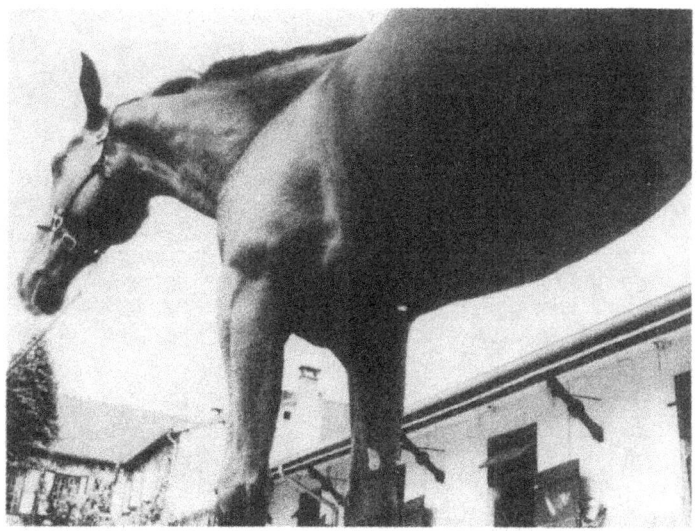

Fig. 25 - Tran Chong

This can be understood, since the spasm observed in an acute crisis is often due mostly to the panic provoked by a feeling of choking. Anxiety is directly linked to the meridian of the stomach, so it is understandable that this meridian plays a part in the process, though the crisis is acted out at the level of the lungs.

To relieve the anxiety linked to the approaching crisis, one should disperse the Energy in the meridian of the stomach thanks to the Li Toe point I have already mentioned, on the coronet above the toe of the hind hoof. It will be useful to add to it the Shu point of the stomach (Wei Shu) in the sixth intercostal space. I would like to remind you that it is to be treated on both sides and that the intercostal spaces have to be counted from rear to front.

Summing up the treatment of the acute crisis of emphysema, you will test, and then massage the Li Toe points on the coronets of the hind hooves, possibly the Shu point of the ninth intercostal space (lung, Fei Shu), then the points of the sixth intercostal space (stomach, Wei Shu), and finally the point of the sternum, Tran Chong.

Chapter 9

WIND SUCKING

Wind sucking is considered by the (French) law as an incurable disease. This legally annuls the sale of a horse if this affliction is detected within the legal time.

Such a horse spends a good part of his time swallowing air, therefore maintaining a chronic inflammation in his stomach. He is a worrier, which is no surprise as we know that with the human there is a link between anxiety, nervous twitches, and gastric pains. The classic "treatment" consists in equipping the horse with a collar which—with or without the help of nails—prevents him from wind sucking by blocking his swallowing. Thus, one opposes the down movement of the pharynx necessary to deglutition; the horse quits wind sucking only because doing so would be too painful. One knows full well that he is not healed, but the bothering symptom was suppressed.

The use of a mechanical device to prevent a horse from swallowing, with the threat of pain to boot, can only increase his anxiety, and foster his gastric pains. Yet this means is not to be disregarded if it allows a horse to better assimilate his food; make no mistake, such a horse assimilates better because his intestinal flora is more balanced in the absence of air and the mucous tissue of his intestine is less irritated, but he is still afflicted with gastritis.

Classical medicine is impotent against gastritis, and horses who wind suck will do so for life, unless they quit of their own, which is exceptional.

Acupuncture can really heal wind suckers, numerous cases show it. It cannot be a chance result since it evidences in the hours following the first session. For a full healing, the first thing to do is to evaluate the basic imbalance of the horse, which is no easy task. On the other hand, one should not expect a thorough healing from only massaging some points. Nevertheless it is certain that one can relieve gastritis and anxiety and even diminish noticeably the frequency of the phenomenon.

The main point to massage is the Shu point of the stomach (Wei Shu, already mentioned) in the sixth intercostal space, which is always sensitive in such a case. Massage it every day, three to four minutes, on both sides. You will reinforce your action by dispersing first the Energy in the meridian of the stomach, through rubbing with a brush the Li Toe point, on the coronet of the hind hooves, above the toe.

Your horse will be less worried, will assimilate his food better, which will allow you to work him more fruitfully.

Chapter 10

HYPERHIDROSIS

This word, although rarely used, designates a very common trouble with the horse. It describes horses who perspire an abnormal amount in relation to the work they do; often these horses will have a second fit of sweat in their stall, though they were dry when entering it. These are horses generally somewhat fearful, who easily make soft droppings and shiver when they are worried. They are prone to diarrhea or spastic colic, rather than colic of stasis (compaction).

This imbalance can be attributed to a predominance of the para-sympathetic nervous system. Its fibers, indeed, have a stimulating effect on most secretions, digestive as well as cutaneous.

One knows in acupuncture that there is some correspondence between the para- sympathetic nervous system and the functions linked to the meridian of the "Three Burners," or "Triple Heater." The Shu point of this meridian is in the fourth intercostal space and is called San Chiao Shu. We have already mentioned it with respect to spasmodic colic and diarrhea.

Daily massage of this point will help your horse, and you will observe that it is very effective for checking an ongoing fit of perspiration.

This method should not be used on a daily basis for drying off a horse who is not afflicted with this unbalance but has been worked somewhat excessively; walking a horse after a working session will always remain useful and is recommended, to facilitate the elimination of muscular toxins as well as on the psychological plane. Anyway, in such case , you will not find any sensitivity with this point and it will be totally inoperative. Perspiration due to working is a natural phenomenon of elimination of part of the toxins released by the effort.

This can be compared to a cyclist swerving to avoid an obstacle. If, with the help of a medication of classical medicine, you block this perspiration, you are going to poison the organism as if you wanted to force the cyclist to run over the obstacle that he has already detected. If, on the other hand, you resort to acupuncture, you won't block anything; it will be as if you contented yourself with warning the cyclist, who will ignore your warning anyway, since he knows where he is going and knows where the real danger lies.

Confronted with hyperhidrosis, classical medicine may have spectacular results, but as long as the animal is under treatment it will be poisoned with toxins, since one of the natural ways of elimination was blocked.

Chapter 11

PAROXYSMAL MYOGLOBINURIA

It is an acute affliction, usually without sequels, but which may have serious and sometimes irreversible consequences if one does not take a few elementary precautions. Before all, one must be capable of diagnosing it and differentiating it from some other afflictions with comparable symptoms.

Its very name is self-explanatory for the essentials if one understands its etymology. "Paroxysmal" means that it is a very intense trouble whose onset is so sudden that it is practically unpredictable.

Myoglobinuria (and not hemoglobinuria, as some often wrongly say) means that one finds myoglobin, which is the principal liquid forming the cells of the fibrous muscles, in the urine of the horse; the urine then takes a brownish red color.

As a matter of fact, it is only occasionally that one has to witness this coloration of the urine, and this for two reasons: on the one hand, the kidneys are irritated by this unexpected product to be eliminated and, for a start, get blocked; on the other hand, the elimination of myoglobin occurs only at an advanced stage of the crisis, which fortunately is rarely attained.

The symptoms come on brutally, always during a working session. The horse stops all of a sudden, in a few strides; he sweats and shivers and above all, he cannot move his hind legs any more. The muscles of his croup become rapidly hard as wood and extremely sore.

Such an incident is explained by the sudden poisoning of muscles overloaded with lactic acid. This is more likely to happen to horses who resume working after a period of rest. The local blood circulation, slowed during the resting period, is not able to rid the muscles of all their toxins and seems overcome by the brusque influx of additional toxins. The rapid development of the crisis is due to a chain reaction like in a nuclear bomb: indeed, when the first muscular fiber tears, it liberates a quantity of lactic acid which, through local irritation, immediately breaks a dozen of other fibers, and so on and so forth. Therefore in a few seconds, there are ten, then a hundred, then a thousand, then ten thousand muscular fibers which are destroyed with a comparable increase in the soreness. Imagine then the sudden influx of lactic acid and cellular waste to the kidneys which are soon incapable of coping with the situation.

When horses were used to pull vehicles, farmers knew this disease very well. It was called the "Monday disease," since it would come up after Sunday's rest. They all knew that they were better off pulling the cart back after unfastening the harness, rather than having the horse walk three or four additional steps forward. Any movement obtained by force could be catastrophic.

You should know that a horse can become irreversibly crippled only by having been brought back forcefully to his stall. The horse, if he refuses to move forward, should be treated on the spot. You may try to encourage him with your voice, to be sure, but above all you should not threaten him with a whip. A really blocked horse can only move his fore legs; his hind legs seem pinned to the ground, so much so that they cross over when the forehand is moved laterally.

Do not mistake this for other cases when a horse refuses to move forward, even if such an error would be less serious than the reverse:

- A horse can refuse to move forward because he is scared, but in this case, if you insist, he will trample in place like the horse who refuses to step into a puddle or to go over a pole on the ground.
- A horse who blocks a stifle does it most often at a halt, and manages to move forward but by dragging his toe on the ground, and swinging his stiffened leg to the outside (he "scythes").

- A horse afflicted with a "sporadic lameness after warming up," due to the presence of a blood clot in the iliac artery, stiffens only one hind leg and continues to move forward, even if he has to keep this limb bent and proceed on three legs. He recuperates totally after a few minutes at a halt and works correctly for some time, before starting to limp again.
- A horse in a bout of acute foundering freezes and refuses to move his front legs. When he moves them, it is by lifting them both together after having engaged his hind legs to an extreme under his body so as to have them carry a maximum of weight. Even if you have to cool constantly his front hooves, you must force him to walk in order to maintain some blood circulation in his feet.
- Finally, a horse hit by tetanus is stiff all over his body, but particularly in his front end; he masticates painfully. It is impossible to be mistaken, since tetanus is a disease accompanied with a "pathognomonic" symptom, i.e., a symptom which is always present and does not show in any other affliction. This symptom alone allows one to affirm that one is in the presence of tetanus, and that it cannot be about something else. This pathognomonic symptom of tetanus is easy to single out: *while* you raise the horse's head by pushing under his chin, the third eyelid falls down all at once, on both sides, covering the whole of the eye. With any sound horse, it moves somewhat. In the case of tetanus, it covers the eye totally and immediately.

A horse who has recurrences of paroxysmal myoglobinuria, or "tying up", which is only its first stage, must be seriously examined at the level of his vertebral column, since it is practically always a slight vertebral blocking which fosters a muscular cramp, which in turn originates the crises.

Your horse being thus blocked, I am proposing to you to relieve him on the spot as you wait for the veterinarian. Waste no time: send for the veterinarian, take off the saddle, and act immediately.

Situated behind the hind leg, the main point is rather sore, but you are not taking any risks, since you set yourself on the side of the horse and above all because the horse is too sore to move his hind legs and try to kick.

This point acts by decongesting the lumbar area and the course of the sciatic nerve. It is situated behind the stifle, in the dip where the big tendon over the hock (the "cord" of the hock) penetrates the back

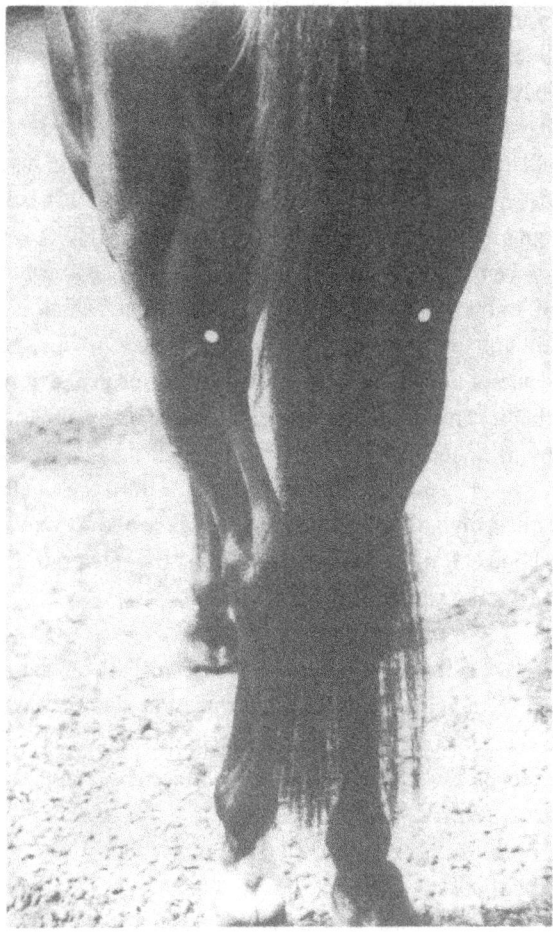

Fig. 26 - Oei Chong

muscles of the leg. Its Chinese name is Oei Chong, a point sovereign for lumbago with the human (Fig. 26).

While positioning yourself on the side of the horse, "hook" your index finger in the dip and massage.

To help the horse urinate and thus get rid of his toxins, massage also the point indicated for urinary retention, the point which helps in opening the neck of the uterus with mares (Prong Kwan Shu). You will be particularly efficient if you massage it while massaging Oei Chong with the other hand, as shown on the picture (Fig. 27). The horse is so incapacitated, and therefore so little dangerous, that you can resort to the help of another person who will do the same on the other side.

A last precaution: if the weather is cold, place a blanket on the loins of the horse.

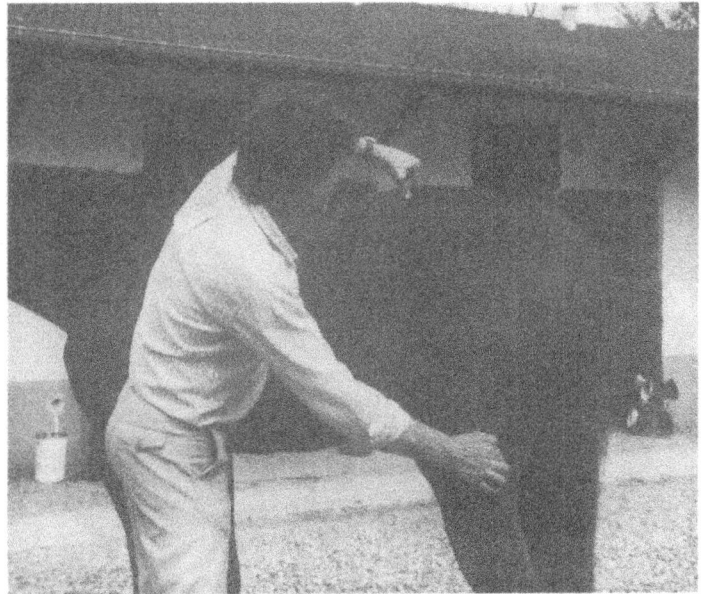

Fig. 27 - Simultaneous Action on Oei Chong and Prong Kwan Shu.

Chapter 12

HEMORRHAGES

As we are, in this book, speaking of pressing and massaging points, it would be too bad to keep silent on an other utilization of this gesture, although it doesn't have anything to do with acupuncture. It is about the manual compression of one or several vessels which are bleeding subsequent to a wound. I will also deal with two cases of hemorrhages when acupuncture can help noticeably; but here are first a few remarks of general interest which I deem useful, since I have seen cases of hemorrhages which well-intentioned persons had worsened out of ignorance.

You should know that in a limb, veins run more superficially and arteries run deeper. Therefore in most cases, it is venous blood which bleeds. The important detail to bear in mind is that, in the veins, the blood runs from the extremity of the limb to the heart, but in spite of that, everybody has the wrong impulse to compress the vein between the heart and the wound. This is the best way to increase the bloodletting!

A compression above the wound has little chances of blocking the main artery, which therefore continues to send blood toward the extremity of the limb, and this blood comes back unopposed to bleed through the ruptured vein, all the more so as the other veins as well are blocked downstream from the wound (above the injury). An ill-applied compression is therefore worse than no compression at all.

Thus one finds compressive bandages which people have endeavored to tighten more in the upper part of the limb and are therefore filled with more blood than the animal would have lost without a bandage!

Before applying a compressive bandage, the wise thing to do is to take the time to search methodically with the finger for the spot where the pressure works best. You will see that with the horse, this spot is often below the wound.

There are two precise cases of hemorrhage where acupuncture certainly helps. Let us examine first the case of a horse who bleeds after castration, or the mare afflicted with a vaginal hemorrhage after foaling (it is about the same points).

All the Chinese documents hold that one just has to plant three needles on the median line of the back, between the spinous processes, from the two last thoracic vertebrae to the two first lumbar vertebrae. It is therefore about the T17-T18, T18-L1, and L1-L2 spaces (Fig. 28).

The action is as strong with a simultaneous massage with three fingers or with transverse rubbing with a brush of the spinal column on this place. The spinous process of the last thoracic vertebra is easily

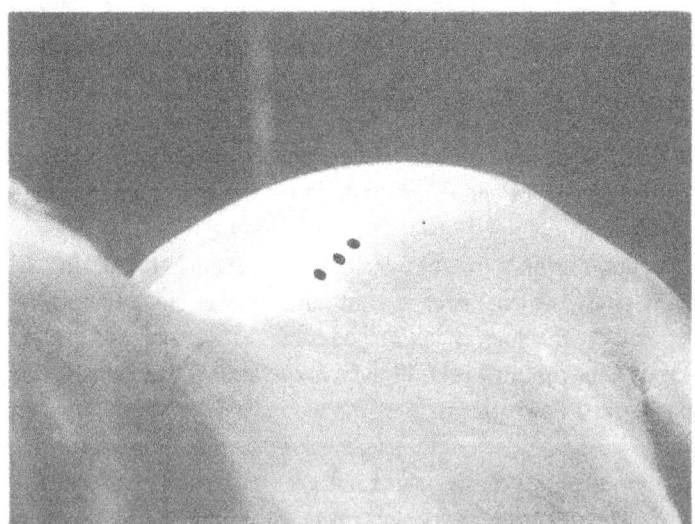

Fig. 28 -Points for vaginal or castration hemorrhage.

spotted by running one's finger along the edge of the last rib.

It seems that the action of these three points is due to two distinct phenomena. Before all, it is a reflex area of the autonomic network in charge of regulating the blood circulation in the areas concerned by the hemorrhages, and on the other hand, these points allow a stimulation of the adrenal glands which, through the discharge of adrenalin, can provoke a vaso-constriction (diminishing the diameter of the blood vessels).

The other case of hemorrhage we are dealing with here is the "epistaxis," which is nothing more than a nosebleed when it proceeds from the nasal mucous or the sinuses, in which case the bleeding generally appears only on one nostril. If the bleeding is bilateral, beware of a possible cardiac problem against which you will not have any recourse, and which necessitates more sophisticated methods of

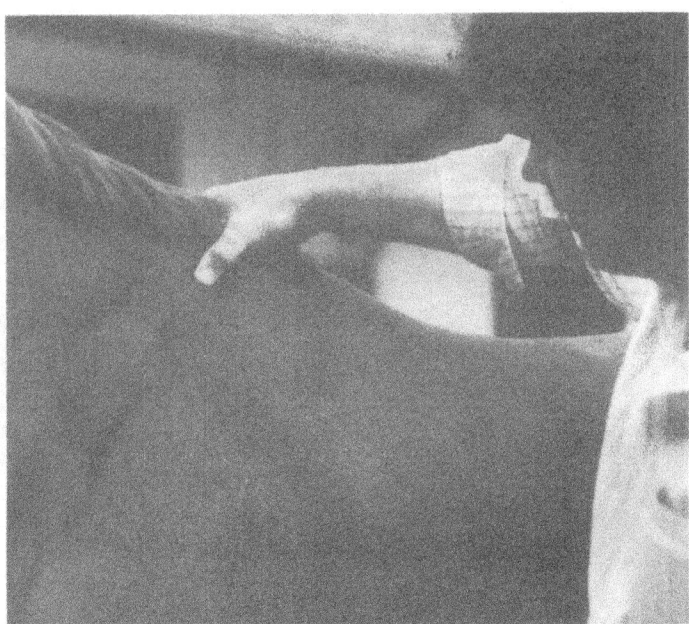

Fig. 29 - Point for epistaxis.

treatment.

The point is bilateral and situated in front of the withers, at the level of the third thoracic vertebra (Fig. 29). As shown on the picture, you can stimulate the point on both sides simultaneously with one hand. The area where this point lies brings in mind the method which consists, with the human, of applying a key or some cold metallic object between the shoulder blades.

Although this point is effectively indicated for epistaxis and gives sometimes obvious results, this time I am less positive than usual, since it is most often rather disappointing. Remember anyway the place of this point, since it will be of another use when we study the set of points indicated for the general relaxation of a horse.

Chapter 13

HEAT STROKE

One should not mistake "heat stroke" with "sunstroke," which is due to the direct action of the sun's rays and which is very rare with the horse whose pigmented skin and tight haired coat protect fairly well from burns by radiation.

Heat stroke may occur outside, in the sun, when there is no breeze, but it is rather an affliction that appears in too hot and above all ill-ventilated enclosures. Think in particular of a horse who waits in a trailer whose vents are shut.

The horse stricken with heat stroke is like drunk, he stumbles along and has violent reactions; it may even be dangerous to saddle him in this state. One must immediately aerate him by getting him out and creating a cool draft. Congestion of the brain is fought by sprinkling skull and ears with cold water.

In addition to these emergency measures, a point of acupuncture brings faster relief to the horse. This point is on the median line, in a crease between the tip of the nose and the base of the nostrils (Fen Shui, Fig. 30).

It is the point which is stimulated by the "twitch," which is often utilized as a means of restraint against rebellious horses. It has been long believed that this device operates only through pain, and through the fear of a greater pain by the slightest movement, but recent studies have shown that the tightening of the twitch provokes in the brain a secretion of endorphine, a hormone close to morphine, with a calming and pain killing action. One sometimes sees horses really going to sleep with a twitch.

It is not surprising that the point of acupuncture situated where the device of restraint works has a calming effect on a congested and aching brain.

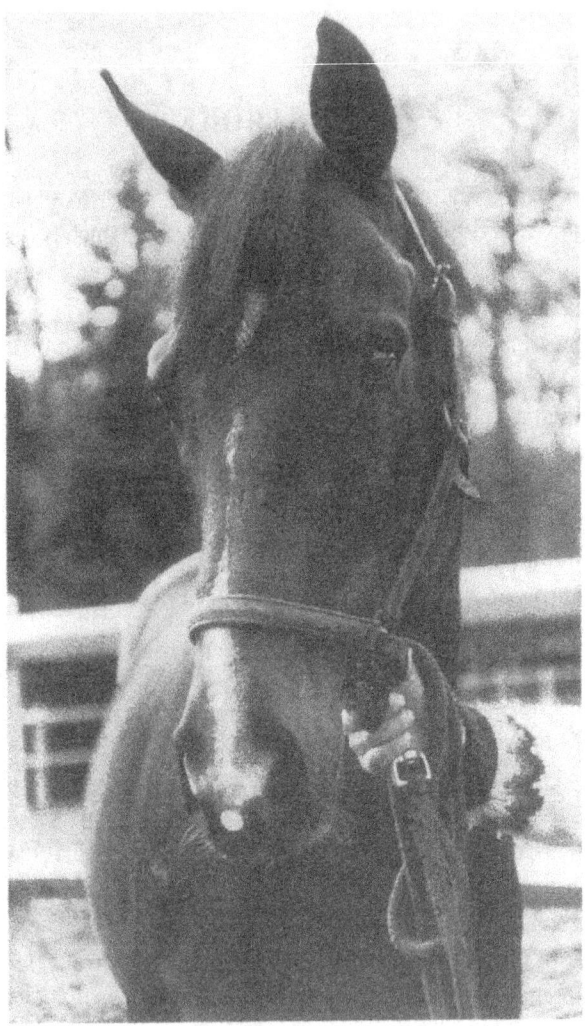

Fig. 30 - Fen Shui

Chapter 14

SHOULDER LAMENESS

For the treatment of lameness in general, refer to the second part of this book which offers a means of alleviating the aches and pains of the locomotive apparatus through basic notions of auriculotherapy.

I am referring first to shoulder lameness because there is an acupuncture point which very easily allows one to know if the shoulder is involved or not, while being very useful as a help for other treatments.

When a shoulder is involved in the lameness, the horse suffers from a neuritis of the branchial plexus, which is comparable to a sciatic inflammation, but for the front limb. The setting of a lameness is often difficult to determine, so the importance of having a test point to tell us whether the shoulder is involved should not be overlooked.

It has been often said, and rightly so, that shoulder lameness is a convenient refuge for imprecise diagnoses. Before deciding that a shoulder is involved when nothing else can be found along the limb, it is important to have the possibility to check it at once. For this, there is a point which reacts very well to the test of pressure in a case of neuritis of the shoulder. It reacts more moderately, but still strongly enough when it is about a pain in the shoulder joint. Anyway, it is concerned only with problems in this area. You should know that even if a lower lesion on the limb can be found and treated, the horse will remain lame as long as the shoulder neuritis has not been taken care of.

You will be in a position to help in the treatment of aches in the shoulder by massaging this point, but only rarely will you reach a complete healing. The relief which you will bring is however useful, but beware: the point is rather sensitive and the horse may try to bite your hand. Yet if your massage is efficient, he will soon calm down.

The effect will be short lived (one working session), because this type of trouble is practically always associated with a blocking of the seventh cervical vertebra. An osteopathic manipulation is then necessary and solves the problem definitively. Other means than osteopathy, as for instance auriculotherapy, may release the vertebral blocking; even a local injection may succeed if it is correctly done at the level of the vertebral joint, and not in the shoulder muscle, but it offers the risk of working only through the pain killing effect, thus allowing the horse to work in spite of the lesion which thenceforth will keep on worsening.

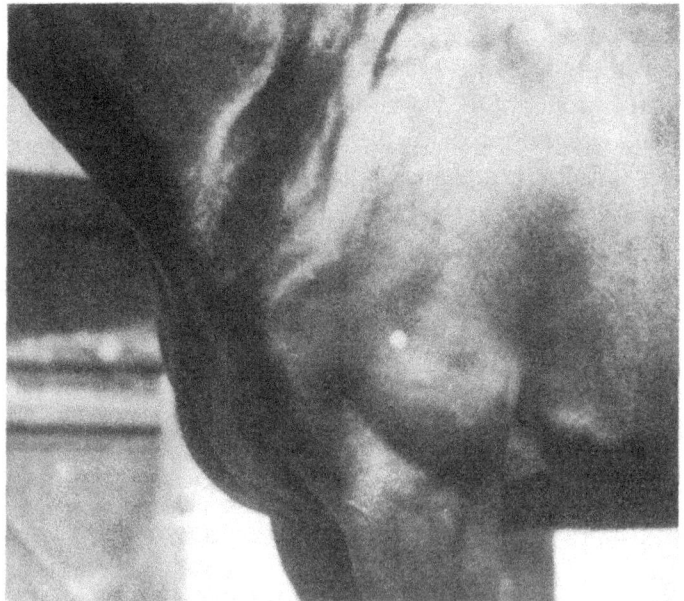

Fig. 31

As I already stated for pulmonary emphysema, anti-inflammatory substances have the big drawback of allowing the horse dangerous movements which otherwise would be impossible due to the pain.

This point, so important for shoulder lameness, and which allows you at least to come up with a more precise diagnosis, is the first point on the lung meridian.

It is called Chong Fu and is situated in the flat part of the shoulder muscles, behind the humerus (Fig. 31). It lies in a depression which is barely visible, but easy to feel with the finger. You will find it three inches back and above the muscular angle where usually the clipping of the coat stops in winter.

As you stick your thumb in this point, pressing somewhat forward, the reaction of the horse will tell you if this shoulder is concerned with the lameness (Fig. 32).

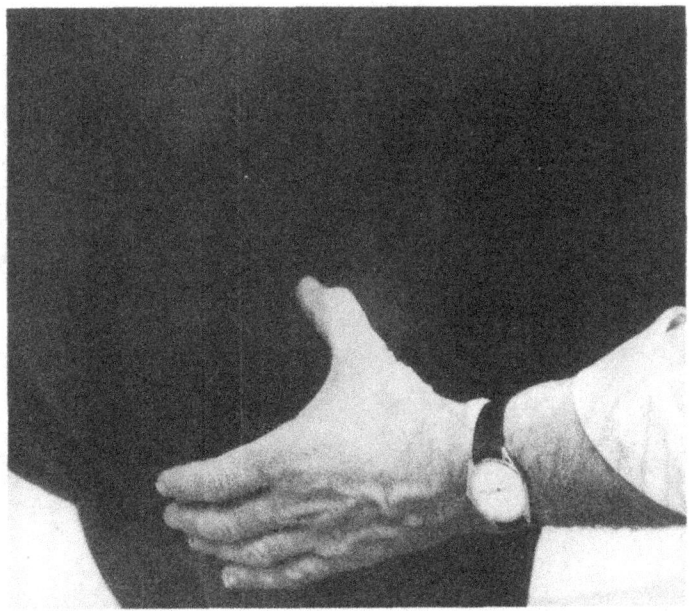

Fig. 32

Finally, I would like to mention that the reaction is positive in the case of elongation or inflammation of the flexors of the limb on the same side (bowed tendon). This is because this lesion is generally linked to a blocking of the seventh cervical vertebra, and that one rarely finds such a tendonitis without a simultaneous neuritis.

This explains the frequent reoccurrences of supposedly healed tendonitis, whereas one overlooked the neuritis. This remark may also be of interest for the human, in particular for many a tennis player.

Chapter 15

AGITATION

Here is a word which is commonly heard amongst horsemen, but few riders seem to be capable of handling their own nervousness. It is easier to cast the blame on a horse, even if horses sometimes have a real talent for unnerving the calmest person!

Agitation is a term which designates many and sometimes quite diverse things, but I think really nervous horses are not as numerous as people say. Many amongst them would rather be calm, but they are somewhat apprehensive (who is not, more or less?), and we give them, knowingly or not, frequent reasons to worry.

Several points are on hand whose stimulation has a calming effect on horses in the real sense of the word, meaning that they give them more confidence when facing a danger, without sedating them.

However, I'd like to say that the most frequent cause for agitation and anxiety with a horse is physical pain. I have seen so many horses become calm and cooperative the moment one found where they were hurting and upon being treated accordingly. We should bear in mind that horses are persuaded that their rider is much stronger than they are. As long as I haven't seen a horse at liberty in a pasture perform half-passes or any other work on his own, with the proper bend, I will remain persuaded that it is psychologic domination which makes equitation possible.

This domination is necessary and makes up for our lack of muscular power. I don't blame it and I am the first to use it when I manipulate the vertebrae of a horse. On the other hand, we should exert it with discretion, since it allows us very easily to make a horse yield even if physical pain is at the origin of his attempts at fighting. Even though accidents are rare, deterioration occurs with numerous horses who are constrained to make movements likely to worsen lesions which we want to ignore. Before overcoming a recalcitrant subject, make sure that he is at that point in time not in pain. The personality of each horse plays a part only as concerns the intensity of the fight, but cases where a problem of submission does not originate in physical pain are very rare. So let's examine how to lessen the agitation of a horse.

I already mentioned the main point (In Tran) in the chapter on foaling (refer to Fig. 16). It is situated between the eyes, on the line of the top of the eyebrows, and you will massage it by spreading your fingers, as if you wanted to elongate it or spread it toward the sides of the forehead. As I also mentioned, the reverse movement would

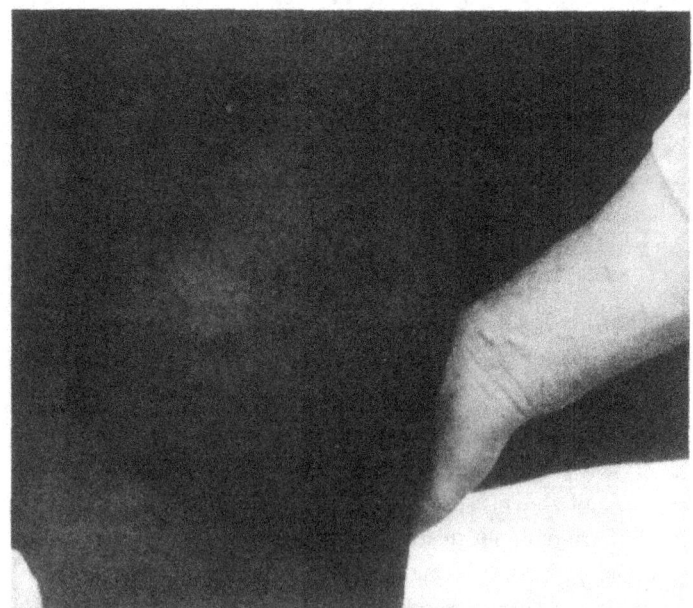

Fig. 33

result in concentrating the horse's attention, hence emphasizing the ongoing problem. This latter way is useful for a distracted horse, who is not focusing on his task.

Another point which plays a part in anxiety is the Shu point of the stomach (Wei Shu, in the sixth intercostal space). As all the other points, it will have some chances working only if it reacts to the pressure test on the horse you are dealing with. I remind you that it is the point for "wind sucking" (refer to Fig. 9).

Other points have a calming effect because they provoke a muscular relaxation and release tightening and tensions due to anxiety. It is, moreover, more about areas than points.

The most important of these areas is the front part of the withers: massage it with full handed grasp while moving the skin longitudinally on the tip of the vertebrae. The horse will raise his head first, then stretch his neck as he twitches his nose, and then you will feel all his body relaxing. This very same massage with the human is well known for bringing a general relaxation and fast well-being.

Another area to know about is that of the last lumbar vertebrae, just before the top of the croup.

The reason why horses are so fond of being massaged inside their elbow joint is that one stimulates in this way a point which disperses the Energy along the meridian of the "triple heater," which is in excess of Energy with the emotional subject (Fig. 33).

You will find other points yourself, proper to the horse you are dealing with, each horse having his likes and dislikes. The relaxation will proceed more from the fact that your horse will understand that you are trying to help him. There is no need to refer to acupuncture to understand that physical contact and caresses will enhance anybody's confidence!

If your relationship with the horse does not limit itself to throwing a saddle on his back straightforward, the complicity between him and yourself while working will develop more easily, and the confidence so obtained will allow you to ask more from him. Only an emotional subject is capable of surpassing himself and doing better than another individual endowed with the same physical capabilities, but first he has to be trusting.

SECOND PART

AURICULOTHERAPY

Chapter 1

To bring relief to cases of lameness and other locomotive problems, we are now going to change our method completely. The mode of treatment will remain manual, but the basic theory will be completely different.

This original therapeutic method can give astounding results with the horse, and deserves our dwelling somewhat on its presumed mode of action and history, if only to pay tribute to Dr. Paul Nogier, the French physician who perfected it.

The Chinese acupuncturists have used for centuries points situated inside the ear, but they would incorporate these points to correspond to the general network of the body. The diagrams of auriculotherapy they publish now do not originate in the tradition, but in Dr. Nogier's works.

As was the case for acupuncture, I am not going to deliver here a course in auriculotherapy, but I will try to explain its principal bases, to the extent where they will allow you to act easily in cases of physical pain which pose real problems to classical medicine.

What I am proposing to you is a simplified utilization of Dr. Nogier's research. Therefore, you will get only a few thorough healings. But on the other hand, as I have observed, you will be able to relieve and put to work horses handicapped with chronic lesions. Besides, you will bring help to the classical treatments of serious afflictions in the locomotive apparatus.

Chapter 2

HISTORIC REVIEW

About 1950, Dr. Paul Nogier had among his patients persons who bore a scar from a burn in the ear, always at the same place. And all would claim that they had had a rebellious sciatic pain treated and healed in this way by a local female healer.

Intrigued and interested, the physician observed that there was always a very sensitive point in the same area with individuals afflicted with a sciatic pain. He then set out to verify if other painful afflictions were linked to a possible point in the ear, and actually found some.

The books he wrote describe in detail his thought process from then on, and I leave it to those interested to refer to them and appreciate his inimitable talent as a narrator. He explains in particular how he noticed that the few points he had detected were distributed rather logically and would practically coincide with the organs and parts of the skeleton of a human fetus in its normal position. Look at an ear, and you will find that it resembles a fetus, the fetus' head being represented by the ear lobe. This similarity was further confirmed when Dr. Nogier localized all the other points, which facilitated his research.

When one pierces little girl's ear lobes, there still remain grandmothers who affirm that this will help them in their sewing, and they are not mistaken since the point of the eye is right in the middle of the lobe. With primitive tribes it is rather the men who have their ears pierced, because they know that in this way they will enjoy a better eyesight for hunting. The traditional earring of the pirates had the same purpose.

In the process of his research, Dr. Nogier established rules of diagnosis and treatment according to his method, and as for what I am proposing to you, here are some important points to keep in mind.

To those familiar with auriculotherapy and its extension which is auriculomedicine, I'd like to point out that I will limit myself here exclusively to what concerns the locomotive apparatus and its afflictions entailing pain. Like in the case of acupuncture, I do not pretend this to be a course, but rather I will indicate a few notions useful to all. Dr. Nogier will not resent me for amputating his method in this way, to the extent that I will perhaps incite a number of individuals to get interested in it and perhaps delve further into it. As far as we are concerned, you should know that:

- To any affliction of the locomotive apparatus (muscles, tendons, skeleton, and joints) involving pain, correspond one or several points of the ear pinna (external part).
- These points are distributed according to a very precise topography which has to be considered for every given specie.
- Spotting the point to be treated can be done in a variety of ways. We will take advantage of it being highly sensitive to pressure. The slight pain induced in this way is very noticeable with respect to the rest of the pinna.
- The possibilities of treatment through this point are manifold (needles, electric current, laser, or even luminous rays projected on a given wavelength, etc.). We will opt for the means of pressing such point for thirty seconds to a minute.
- Although with this simplified technique the response is sometimes immediate, one must nevertheless maintain its effect through one or two additional daily sessions for a few days.
- In most cases, with the horse, the point to work is found on the same side as the affliction. If you are positive about the location of the trouble and cannot find the point where it should be, try the

other ear; but such cases are rare. Rather, make sure that you have searched correctly where you should have.

• The sensitivity of the point diminishes in the progress of the sessions. There will, however, remain a slight reaction after the possible healing, if the affliction has left a definitive, although non-hurting, lesion (a scar, callosity of fracture, bony growth).

Chapter 3

MODE OF ACTION

To better understand the limits of your action, it may be useful to know, at least succinctly, how these gestures can have a therapeutic effect.

In a living organism, any trouble is reported via complex circuits to that extraordinary computer which is the brain, so as to enable it to react accordingly and try to restore the proper order. One knows that, depending on the place of the body which is concerned, a specific area of the brain will receive the information.

From this center which receives the alarm, the brain will send orders to organize a set of measures necessary to safeguard and restore. These measures are sometimes excessive, all the more as the sharp pain at the origin of the process leaves a mark harmful to the nervous system by weakening the cells which received the initial information. This trace may then maintain a reaction no longer necessary. This explains, for instance, why the edema subsequent to a sprain lasts so long or why an ancient fracture can hurt long after the healing of the bone.

It is believed that the point of auriculotherapy is projected in the brain exactly at the same place as the area of the body (joint or other) which corresponds to it.

All happens as if stimulating the point does erase the trace left by the corresponding trouble in the nervous cells. The brain then "forgets" the event which had attracted its attention and quits minding it; more particularly, the pain disappears rapidly.

If the aggression was only temporary (sprain), auriculotherapy brings a fast healing. On the other hand, if the aggression lasts, as in the case of a microbial arthritis, this latter "cries" so strongly about its problem that the treatment can only limit the response of brain and then keep it just at the appropriate level for it to be effective without spawning new troubles until complete healing.

Such a mode of action brings to mind an unfortunately frequent practice which classical veterinary medicine uses to "heal" some cases of lameness of the horse: denervation.

This surgical intervention, which consists of severing the nerves in the limb where the trouble lies, suppresses the information destined to the brain and prevents it from reacting; but this action is blind and definitive. A horse having undergone such an operation is no longer lame, but if he gets a nail stuck in his foot, he will not feel it, nor will he signal if his prior affliction worsens, unless his lesions spread toward new territories whose nerves have been spared. In addition, and above all, his brain can no longer regulate the blood circulation proportional to his work. A wooden leg is certainly less likely to develop corns!

Auriculotherapy therefore has nothing to do with this barbarian procedure which in fact is a renouncing of medicine.

The method of treatment which derives from it and that I am proposing to you is very simple but somewhat delicate to implement since it acts by provoking a pain; moreover, horses do not like much to have their ears tinkered with. One may sometimes hate to use a twitch, but one should resort to such an extreme measure only when one is positive about the point and its indication.

Chapter 4

TOPOGRAPHY

While the map of the human ear is perfectly known, that of the animals is far from being established. After a few years of tests on obvious cases, I can propose to you a map which is certainly not completely faithful to reality, but whose utilization is satisfactory enough for it to be considered as a starting base. It must be verified and refined, and every person who practices this method of treatment can easily help by contributing their personal observations.

The pinna of a horse's ear is far from suggesting any kind of fetus! I therefore have searched, on the dog first, referring to the human topography, after having established that the points are linked to the folds of the cartilage which bear the same name with both species.

The map established little by little on the dog yields indisputable results, although sometimes difficult to explain through the classical reasoning. Joint pains, as for instance the degenerative osteochondritis of the shoulder, disappear very easily in this way. It seems incredible that a dog's lameness due to a rupture of the crossed ligament of the knee may heal in eight to ten days after a clip was fixed on a point of the ear! A dozen cases have already shown it, including that of a one hundred and eighty seven pound mastiff.

For those who have a dog, and a ballpoint pen to press on the points, here is the map of the canine ear (Fig. 34). Perhaps you won't get as good results as you would with a clip or laser beam, but you will be pleasantly surprised by the results anyway.

The topography of the horse is more vague (Fig. 35). Actually, it were only areas and a few more precise points that allowed me to establish a tentative scheme. The points on the lower extremity of the limbs are localized well enough to be useful if one considers the great number of cases of lameness on the horse's lower legs.

The confirmed zones are in bold lines, the dotted lines indicate deductions that must be confirmed or unconfirmed by subsequent trials and research.

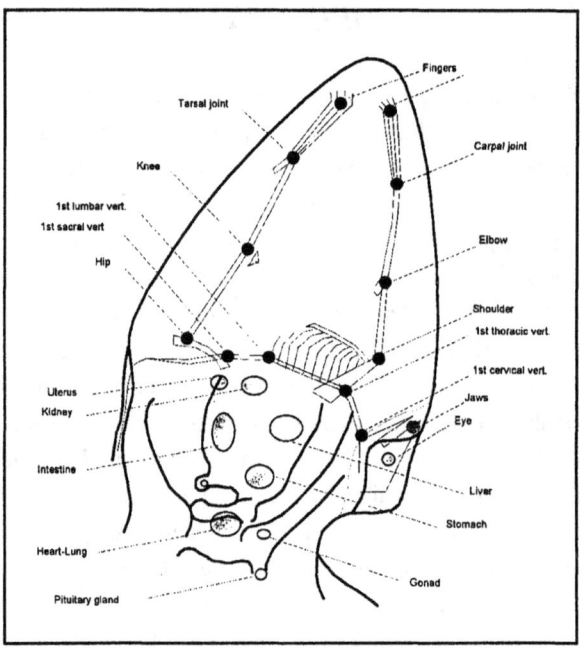

Fig. 34 - Left ear acupuncture points in the dog, according to Dr. Dominique Giniaux.

MAP OF THE LEFT EAR OF THE DOG

With the dog as with the human, one finds the point and treats it very easily with the tip of a ballpoint pen. The reaction of defense of the animal is noticeable with respect to the neighboring points; it is advisable to muzzle the dog with a cord.

Notice that the troubles concerning the forelegs of a dog cannot be treated in this way if his ears have been bobbed.

The map of the cat is similar, but the area corresponding to the front leg is spread over a larger surface (retractile claws, and more complex movements).

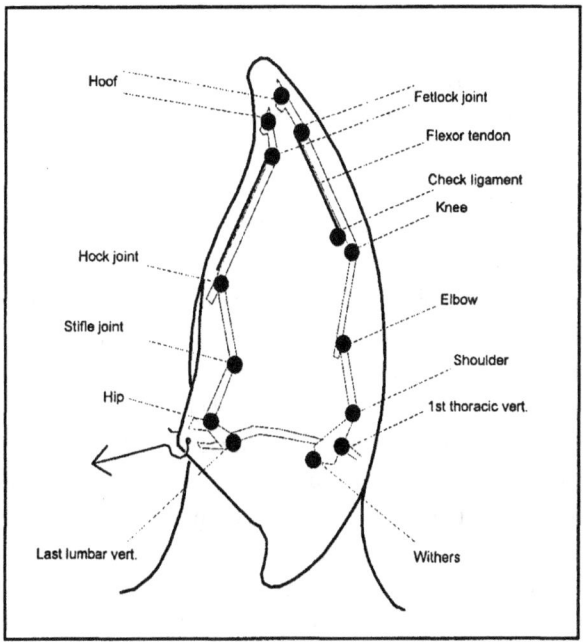

Fig. 35 - Left ear acupuncture points in a horse, according to Dr. Dominique Giniaux.

MAP OF THE LEFT EAR OF THE HORSE

The area with dotted lines must be established more precisely, by referring to the cartilaginous folds one feels in the pinna.

The actual state of research is not very advanced, but it already allows one to localize points of great utility for the lameness in the horse's lower legs.

Please note that the fore limb projects itself along the *rear* edge of the ear. With some training, you will be able to determine the level of a lameness as accurately as with the method of sequential nerve blocking. On the other hand, a nail is too coarse a tool to distinguish a bony growth on a canon bone from a tendinous lesion at the same level. This nuance bears little significance since one brings a relief anyway, but it is essential for assessing the risks involved with the resumption of work. A tendon where the pain was reduced heals faster, but remains very fragile as long as its fibers are not repaired.

In the realm of tendinitis and "bowed tendons," it is absolutely undeniable that auriculotherapy works and complements quite fairly the classical treatments. Some navicular diseases are markedly relieved, and one must do one's best for the development of such a therapeutic tool.

The area of the stifle is still not well enough explored, yet it would be very useful. I am thinking of the nasty problem of blocking of a patella which could very well be treated in this way, but I cannot be more affirmative without a number of tests and proofs.

One may see on the map that the horse's limbs are a linear and very narrow surface, which simplifies the use of the method. The surface of projection of the diverse parts of the body seems to be linked to the importance of the innervation in each area. With the human, the hand is much innervated, as much for its possibilities of complex movements, as for its very refined faculties of palpation. It occupies a great surface in the ear with respect to the rest of the body.

The horse's limbs make only simple movements, always on the same plane, and their use in the domain of palpation is limited to knowing whether they touch the ground or not. It therefore is not surprising that a line of points suffices to represent their importance for the nervous system. Another proof for this theory is that the projection of the front paw of a cat is proportionally wider than of a dog: this is consistent with the type of claws, the gestures of grooming oneself, hunting, etc.

Chapter 5

TECHNIQUE

The very same gesture will allow you to determine the point and treat it. For the lower part of both legs, the line is parallel to the edge of the pinna; the distance from the edge varies according to the subject, but this won't bother us since it is about a line and there are no points outside it.

The nail of the thumb, placed perpendicularly to the line, is going to look for and find the point through successive pressures while moving carefully along the line. The pressure should be rather light and above all as even as possible throughout the whole process of exploring the line point by point.

When you spot a more sensitive point, continue further beyond it in order to verify that the sensitivity is lesser elsewhere, and then come back to the point where the horse reacts.

Then proceed to the treatment by pressing your nail stronger and stronger, although without making the horse jump, in which case his ear would escape your hand anyway. Maintain the pressure to a bearable intensity for about one minute.

It is sometimes more efficient to modulate the pressure through alternate pressures without interrupting the contact with the skin. As we do so, we may observe that the point becomes less and less sensitive and that this improvement is linked to the improvement of the affliction we try to treat.

For the left side of the horse, hold the base of his ear with your left hand while you mask his eye with your left front arm, and search with the right hand and right thumbnail. For the other side, left handed persons have an advantage; right handed persons have more difficulties masking the horse's eye, since it is the right arm, active at this moment, which must try to do it. This is an important remark since the horse is less worried if he does not see the hand which moves.

If you experience difficulties in the beginning or if the horse does not stand this kind of investigation, don't get nervous and chew on your nails. If only because without nails, you could not treat the horse anymore! This is only half a joke: bear in mind that nervousness in all its forms is detrimental when dealing with a horse.

This technique based on auriculotherapy must be accompanied with a few precautions.

- To start with, one must know the map, at the present stage of our knowledge of it, so as to have to search only a limited area. If one searches everywhere rapidly and at once, one irritates the ear enough for its sensitivity to lose any meaning and one will have to pause before starting again, which the horse will not appreciate.
- It is not rare that one finds two points for only one trouble: in addition to the point corresponding to the lesion, there is often a positive response at the level of the projection of the sector of the vertebral column wherefrom the nerves involved in the diseased member originate.

There is here an obvious link with osteopathy which establishes a participation of the spinal column to all peripheral problems. The vertebrae are not incriminated. They can be blocked because of the peripheral trouble, as well as the other way around. This particular form of medicine which is thoroughly in accord with the laws of acupuncture and auriculotherapy deserves a book for itself.[1]

- Be wary of too rapid results which this technique will sometimes bring about; they do not inevitably mean that the real healing took place.

I explained in the lines above that one acts by lifting up the threshold of response on the cells traumatized by the original event.

If tissues were damaged, they could not heal as fast as the pain was yielding, and a new request during the work will send such a signal that the threshold will lower anew, allowing the harmful influxes to reach the brain.

Therefore remember well that it is not because a tendon has retrieved its normal appearance that it is completely healed. For the same reason many have been disappointed by the laser treatment of tendinitis.

The laser beam, on the appropriate frequency, drains perfectly the tendinous lesion and therefore facilitates a faster restoration of the fibers, but this restoration requires anyway some time. Too many people believe that it is about a problem of power of the laser beam. One witnesses nowadays a real armament race. Everyone wants the bigger (and by the same token more expensive) laser. I have been able

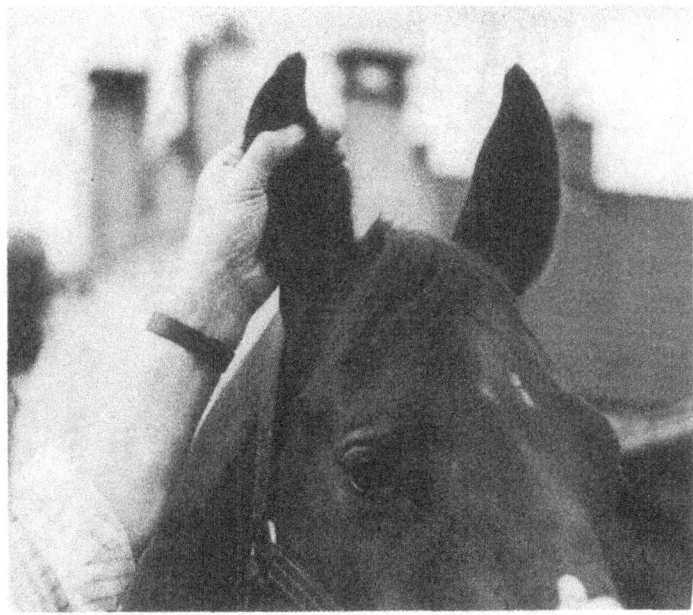

Fig. 36 - Point of the right hock

to establish that a small laser, working on batteries, which one can handle with one hand, is as efficient if one knows which frequencies to use for the case of the individual in question.

Using powerful lasers is sometimes tantamount to trying to kill a fly with an artillery gun, whereas a simple swatter would have done the job!

While it is true that a big laser sometimes dissipates better the local edema, it does not heal the lesion faster than a small one whose frequency is well adjusted; it therefore has the drawback of making one believe too early that the heeling is complete.

The only method which has shown me so far that it is possible to really shorten the period of healing of a bowed tendon is the auriculomedicine associated with the appropriate osteopathic manipulations. I have been in a position to verify it several times, notably with

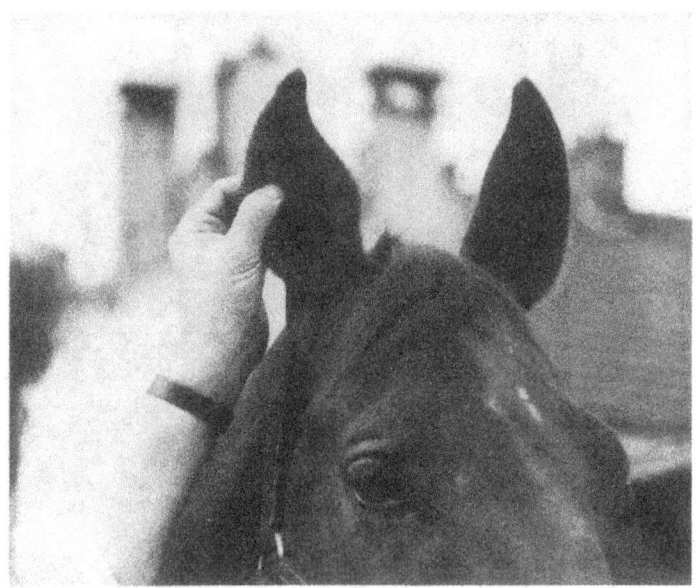

Fig. 37 - Point of the right elbow

a famous galloper.

Auriculomedicine is the evolved form of auriculotherapy; it allows one, by way of the ear, to re-equilibrate the circulation of the Energy in the whole of a perturbed organism. The study of its techniques exceeds by far the limits of the present treatise.

Coming back to a simplified utilization of auriculotherapy, bite the bullet and make trials on the basis of the points already known for the lower extremity of the limbs. You will progressively refine your technique and set out to determine other points. Progress will result only from the collection of a maximum number of experiments which will allow a permanent reorganization of the horse's ear topography.

If you are interested in this work, do it seriously and systematically. Check carefully before affirming anything on the basis of only one case, and don't forget to check that there is not a nail in your horse's hoof before trying treating his lameness through auriculotherapy!

Try to keep a critical judgement versus what you think you have discovered. Enthusiasm should not obliterate common sense. "Each time that we try to give a solution of a problem, we should also try as rigorously as possible to go beyond it, rather than defending it." (Karl R. Popper in **The Logic of Scientific Discovery.**)

[1] This book **Les Chevaux m'ont dit**, published in France by Favre, was subsequently written by Dr. Giniaux. Its English translation by Jean-Claude Racinet was published in 1997 under the title **What the Horse Have Told Me** by Xenophon Press.

Chapter 6

CONCLUSION

The pieces of advice I have put together in this book are only a starting point, but they open doors onto a fascinating domain. A reflex action of the "Shu" points is perfectly comprehensible in Western medicine since the latter acknowledges the role of the autonomic nervous system, whose centers are directly connected to these points. By contrast, it seems more surprising to trigger off the coming up of the milk with a mare by stimulating points at the hock, or that two points in the ear may concern respectively the two extremities of the horse (front legs and back legs phalanges).

Upon establishing the reality of these facts, one cannot deny any longer the action of acupuncture. Even if, out of a personal choice, one prefers to stick to Western medicine, one knows that there exist other ways, as worthwhile, and one will not refuse systematically to resort to them if they look more indicated for some cases.

My main purpose would be fulfilled if I had awakened the interest of a sufficient number of persons. It is about time to quit the stage of today's lingering discussions aimed at persuading narrow minds by using narrow examples. Let us go beyond the kind of popularization books like "A few amusing experiments of physics." Our goal is not to persuade systematic critics whose only motive is that they don't like to be intellectually challenged. I shall have reached my goal if some of my readers understand that it is important to proceed in this direction, and to partake in this effort themselves.

One can distinguish nowadays two different currents in acupuncture research: the first is made by those who try to use it as best as they can while refining their practice and the comprehension of the traditional laws; the other consists in a fundamental research which is more satisfying for Western minds. The latter want before all to set in evidence the reality of the pathways of Energy which have been transmitted to us and understand the physiological process of their mode of action.

Fundamental research is indispensable to the progress of Science, hence of Humanity, and I don't deny the foremost interest in such an endeavor. But I think that it won't help in utilizing the art of acupuncture. Geniuses were needed in the research which led to television, but obviously we should not ask them to fix our television set. Likewise, the best orchestra conductors know the rules of harmony and the nuances they can expect from each of their instrumentalists, but they could not manufacture the instruments their musicians are using.

Setting in evidence specific cells at the level of the acupuncture points is not what will create better acupuncturists, although such a discovery would be undeniably fascinating.

By contrast, one can hold that any progress in the Art of harmonizing all the pathways of Energy in an organism, and therefore in the practice of acupuncture or related medicines using its traditional laws, will profit all kinds of patients, horses, or others.

These medicines are not merely a different way to heal, they constitute a more universal approach to what a balanced living organism should be.

While broadening the scale of the therapeutic possibilities, which should remain the main incentive, these modes of reasoning will allow one to consider from a new angle the functioning of the Universe as well as the rapport between individuals or societies.

And what is the goal of a true horseperson, if not trying to better understand all the refinements in the rapport between two individuals in the seeking of harmony?

SUMMARY CHART

Affliction	Point	Locality
Impaction colic	Ta Shang Shu	Between 18th and 17th rib, on the edge of the common dorso-lumbar muscular mass. Bilateral.
	Tsian Shu	Hollow of the right side, between point of the hip and the 18th rib. Unilateral.
	Pi Shu	Between 16th and 15th rib (third space). Edge of the common muscular mass. Bilateral.
	Yun Men	Lowest point of the belly, three to four inches from medial line. Bilateral.
Gastric colic	Wei Shu	Between 13th and 12th rib (sixth space). Edge of the common muscular mass. Bilateral.
Spasmodic colic	Hsiao Shang Shu	Between second and third lumbar. Mid distance between spine and common mass. Bilateral.
	San Shiao Shu	Between 15th and 14th rib (fourth space). Edge of common muscular mass. Bilateral.
	Pi Shu	See Impaction colic.
	Yun Men	See Impaction colic.
Diarrhea	Tien Shu	On the cowlick between umbilicus and stifle. Bilateral.

Affliction	Point	Locality
	Hsiao Shang Shu	See Spasmodic colic.
	San Shiao Shu	See Spasmodic colic.
Urinary colic	Prang Kwan Shu	Between sixth lumbar and sacrum (last hollow between spinal column and pelvis). Two and a half to three and a half inches from medial line. Bilateral.
Urinary retention in a trailer	Ibid.	Ibid.
Difficult foaling	In Tran	Forehead, between the eyebrows, middle point.
	Ko Shu	Between 11th and 10th rib (eight space). Edge of common muscular mass. Bilateral.
	Prang Kwan Shu	See Urinary colic.
Coming up of milk:		
Painful (excess)	Li Toe	Front part of hind legs coronet. Bilateral.
Insufficient	Tsie Tsri	Front crease of hock, outside of extensor tendon. Bilateral.
Foaling:		
Apnea	Ren Chong	Middle of the tip of the nose, over the lip.
Choking	Roe Yin	Perineum, under the anus.

Affliction	Point	Locality
Retention of meconium	Kwan Yuan	Between umbilicus and pubis. Middle.
Retention of placenta	"Sacral holes"	On the croup, lateral edges of sacrum. Bilateral.
	Prang Kwan Shu	See Urinary colic.
Emphysema	Fei Shu	Between 10th and 9th rib (ninth space). Edge of common mass. Bilateral.
	Tran Chong	Hollow, under the sternum. Middle line.
	Wei Shu	See Gastric colic.
	Li Toe	See excessive coming up of milk.
Wind sucking	Wei Shu	See Gastric colic.
Hyperhidrosis	San Shiao Shu	See Spasmodic colic.
Myoglobinurea	Oei Chong	Behind the hind leg, in the dip at the level of stifle, where thick ligament blends into muscle. Bilateral.
	Prang Kwan Shu	See Urinary colic. Work simultaneously with Oei Chong. Bilateral.
Hemorrhage (castration)	Twan Tsie	Dorsal line. Spaces T17 - T18, T18 - L1, L1 - L2. Middle.
Epistaxis (nose bleading)	"Withers"	One and a half to two inches under top line of withers. Bilateral.

Affliction	Point	Locality
Heat stroke	Fen Shui	Above tip of nose, right below the bottom line of nostrils. Middle.
Neuritis of shoulder	Chong Fu	Lateral face of shoulder. Where dorsal (top) edge of humerus intersects with medial line of front leg. Bilateral.
Agitation	In Tran	See Foaling.
	Wei Shu	See Gastric colic.
	"Withers"	Like with epistaxis, but with a full-handed movement of the skin. Bilateral.
	"Elbow"	Under arm pit, rubbing the inside of elbow. Bilateral.
Auriculotherapy: Pains in the loco-		

www.ingramcontent.com/pod-product-compliance
Lightning Source LLC
Chambersburg PA
CBHW050600300426
44112CB00013B/1999